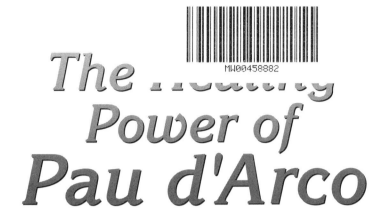

# The Healing Power of Pau d'Arco

The Divine Tree of the South American Shamans
Provides Extraordinary Healing Benefits

*Translated by Christine M. Grimm*

LOTUS LIGHT
SHANGRI-LA

1st English edition 1998
© by Lotus Light Publications
   Box 325, Twin Lakes, WI 53181
The Shangri-La Series is published in cooperation
with Schneelöwe Verlagsberatung, Federal Republic of Germany
© 1997 reserved by the Windpferd Verlagsgesellschaft mbH, Aitrang
All rights reserved
Translated by Christine M. Grimm
Cover design by Kuhn Grafik, Digitales Design, Zurich
Illustrations: Aladin's Bookdesign, S. 20: Okapia
Composition and make-up: *panta rhei!* – MediaService Uwe Hiltmann
Production: Schneelöwe, D-87648 Aitrang

ISBN 0-914955-52-7
Library of Congress Catalogue No. 97-78481

Printed in the USA

# The Healing
## Power of
# Pau d'Arco

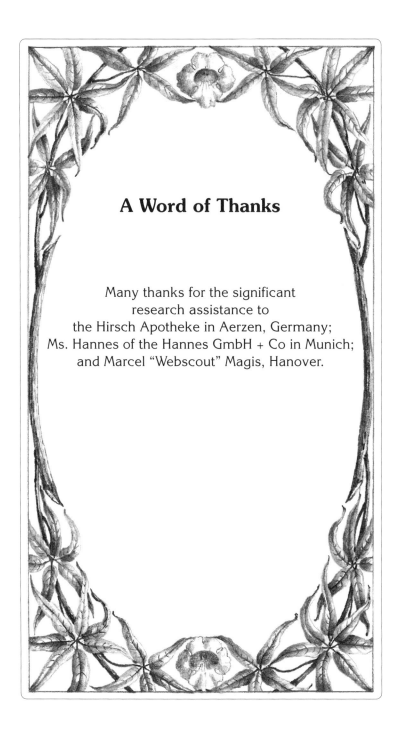

# A Word of Thanks

Many thanks for the significant
research assistance to
the Hirsch Apotheke in Aerzen, Germany;
Ms. Hannes of the Hannes GmbH + Co in Munich;
and Marcel "Webscout" Magis, Hanover.

# Table of Contents

# Preface

The research for this book was done with the greatest possible accuracy and care, and attention has been paid to the most recent status of research in the preparation of the text. However, neither the author nor the publisher shall assume any form of liability for the validity of the information in this book.

The author and publisher expressly recommend that you consult a competent medical professional for the treatment of all health disorders and also discuss with him or her the use of pau d'arco tea and catuaba tea, as well as any other food supplements, health-promoting foods, and the corresponding applications mentioned in this book.

In no way should the information in this book be understood as an invitation to self-medication for diseases requiring treatment. Doctors, healing practitioners, and pharmacists can give professionally competent information for individual application, the general suitability, means of application, and appropriate dosage for the health-improving aids specified in this book. They should definitely be consulted before using such remedies.

# Introduction

## How Pau d'Arco Tea Found Me

The first time I heard of pau d'arco tea was in the year 1995 on a television talk show about methods of alternative healing. A healing practitioner spoke about a hay fever therapy that he had developed and mentioned that he additionally prescribed pau d'arco tea for his patients on a regular basis. This medicinal plant was not only very effective but also tasted good. Unfortunately, the topic changed rather rapidly and I learned nothing more about it. However, I had become curious—a particularly healing herbal tea that was even said to have an acceptable aroma. Hmm!

Unfortunately, as so often happens in my days filled with many interesting events, I initially skipped over p

Unfortunately, as so often happens in my days filled with many interesting events, I initially skipped over pau d'arco and forgot that I actually wanted to start researching it. But as "coincidence" would have it, during the course of the next few months I heard about this mysterious medicine tea time and again from various sources.

As is my practice when I want to learn more about something, I reserved a few days for research and went on expeditions through libraries and bookstores. Then I questioned many of the healing practitioners and naturopathically oriented doctors with whom I'm personally acquainted. However, I couldn't find out more concrete information than: "It's probably a medicinal plant from the rainforests of South America. It's good against cancer, tumors remit, and symptoms triggered by cancer quickly disappear; disease-causing fungi in the body, like *Candida*, are killed; and pau d'arco makes a very effective contribution to general detoxification. At the same time, it's completely harmless and has a very good taste. It's quite delicious! How does it have this effect?

No idea. A patient/colleague/friend of mine recommended it to me. I simply tried it out and it helps wonderfully."

The results weren't very satisfying. In addition, I had in the meantime discovered through my own experience that pau d'arco tea tastes very good: like vanilla, a bit like cinnamon, and pleasantly smoky. I discovered it at my tea shop around the corner. Since then, I've been drinking it on a regular basis since I like the taste and the tea is good for me. It was quite interesting to read some information that the owner of the tea shop had compiled himself and the friendly saleswoman handed to me along with the package of tea, without even being asked for it. Here I could read that pau d'arco has been sold for 80 years by Viking traders in Europe. Even at that time, it was widely praised by herbalists because of its great healing power and could only be exchanged for gemstones. Furthermore, it has been proved that a Russian czar lived to be 130 years old and enjoyed at least one cup of pau d'arco every day. His name wasn't mentioned. "Well," I thought to myself, "there are many stories that can be told." Still, if this story should have some truth to it ...

During a longer telephone conversation, my tea dealer mentioned that pau d'arco tea was being prescribed by many doctors working with naturopathic methods in the area. He had actually included it in his program because of the constant demand for it—and the tea was selling very well. A few days later, while enjoying a cappuccino and an antipasto plate lovingly put together by Mama Lena, the friendly owner of my favorite Italian bistro, I thought about how I could get more information about the "miracle tea." There hadn't yet been any books published about it in Germany. I sent a quick prayer to heaven that if someone up there thought that pau d'arco was important for me, I should get the message. Then I pulled a computer journal just purchased at the newspaper store next door out of my briefcase and opened it randomly. "Research in the Internet" stood printed in bold type at the top of the page. "How you can get the most up-to-date information on any topic through the World Wide Web, the global computer network." I was astonished and read the ads, which convinced me: If there would be any extensive information at all anywhere about the miracle herb from the jungles of South America, then it would be in the Internet.

The hunting fever had hit me once again. A few hours and a great many phone calls later, one of my friends had revealed himself to be an Internet surfer. He was enthusiastic about me finally bringing him a serious, useful assignment in the World Wide Web and gladly agreed to browse through the Internet to look for information about pau d'arco for me.

I didn't have to wait long for the results. In the course of the next week, time and again I received disks packed full of reports, the latest research results, and bibliographical references. When I had read these initial texts on the monitor of my computer, I knew that the entire effort had been worth it ...

Pau d'arco, called the "divine tree" by the Indios of South America, is one of the most effective, economical, and versatile remedies against a multitude of acute and chronic diseases that has ever been discovered. It quickly became clear to me that this knowledge had to be made available to as many people as possible. My decision to write a book about pau d'arco had become definite.

And now you hold the results in your hands. I wish you many pleasant hours of reading and am certain that you will be just as enthusiastic about pau d'arco as I am.

Walter Lübeck

# Chapter 1

# This Is Pau d'Arco Tea

Pau d'arco tea consists of the inner bark of the lapacho tree, which is peeled and rasped one to two times a year. This finely cut, quite soft "young wood" is offered as loose tea or in tea bags.

The lapacho tree, which has the botanical name of Tabebuia avellanedae or Tabebuia impetiginosa, grows in wide areas of South America and Central America. These include Argentina, Bolivia, Brazil, Columbia, Ecuador, French Guinea, Paraguay, Peru, Surinam, Trinidad, Tobago, and Venezuela. There are dozens of regional subspecies of this plant.* It can adapt to various environmental conditions, is robust, and relatively undemanding.

The family name of "Tabebuia" comes from an Indio language spoken by various tribes in Brazil. Some native tribes call the tree "ant wood" (taheebo) since ants like to nest in its trunk when it dies. As an aside, the tree isn't directly infested by termites, ants, and other parasites while it's alive. The wood is enormously hard, robust, and resistant, which is why people have liked to use it for making bows, among other things, since the time o the ancient Incas. For this reason, wood experts also call it the "South American Oak" and the lapacho tree is commonly called pau d'arco (bow tree). In addition, it contains substances that kill vermin or make life unpleasant for them. The name of the species "impetiginosa" was derived from the traditional custom of using the bark tea against the disease impetigo, an inflammation of the facial skin accompanied by suppuration.

---

* There are about six variations in Central America, more than 70 in the Caribbean, and more than 20 in South America.

## Digression: Is The South American Rainforest Endangered By The Use Of Pau D'Arco Tea?

Based on all the information that I've gathered, I can say a clear "no!" to this question. The inner bark of the lapacho tree is, similar to the cork oak, harvested in such a way as to leave the tree in a state of complete health. In addition, there is an entire series of lapacho farms where the trees grow by means of controlled, organic cultivation. The bark harvest is carried out once a year on the wild-growing trees and twice a year on plantations. However, the best lapacho quality originates from the wild harvest since the complete combination of active ingredients (in the optimal composition) can only be found at an age of about 40 years. Since the extensive medicinal use of pau d'arco only began one or two decades ago, the trees of most plantations aren't old enough to be able to deliver the best quality of pau d'arco tea. But this situation is improving from year to year. And since the majority of the lapacho plantations have decided on organic-ecological cultivation right from the start, they are providing a contribution to environmentally friendly agriculture and ecologically meaningful jobs that shouldn't be underestimated. At the same time, this largely corresponds with the traditional culture of the Indios.

The industrial use of lapacho wood also creates bark, which is offered as tea. However, this source appears to play an increasingly minor role on the market. The harvest of pau d'arco tea therefore definitely doesn't endanger the existence of this type of tree.

But the situation is different for the industrial exploitation of lapacho wood, which is beautiful and tremendously stable in mechanical terms. Although the genus "Tabebuia" is widespread throughout South America and even, according to the latest reports by independent environmental organizations, far from extinction, some few regional subspecies are terribly endangered. This is why the development of lapacho plantations and the use of the tea is so important in order to secure its existence for the long term. More on this in the following section.

# Lapacho—A Popular Timber

Lapacho provides a very stable and decorative wood and has long been used for a great variety of purposes as a result. For example, as parquet floor, for radio and television cabinets, furniture, and ship planks. The lapacho tree has been used as a timber for many purposes by industry because of its outstanding mechanical and aesthetic qualities. The lapacho is definitely not threatened by extinction and is widespread in large regions of South America, to an extent comparable with the fir tree in Germany. It can be found both in the rainforests and lowland plains, as well as in the mountains up to an elevation of about 4,000 meters above sea level. It grows on good topsoil, in the moist jungle of the Amazon region, but is just as satisfied with a rather sandy subsoil. The botanic genus Tabebuia includes about 100 species, which are distinguished from each other after the appearance of the leaves and flowers. The lapacho with its many regional subspecies occurs as a bush, but also as a tree. Fully grown, the tree reaches a height of up to 25 meters and achieves a maximum trunk diameter of 75 centimeters. Under good conditions, it can grow to be a proud 700 years old.

Only after about the 40th year of life can the valuable substances be found in full concentration and optimal composition, which is the basis of its outstanding medicinal power, in the inner bark. The trunk is usually very straight and, measured from the ground, free of twigs for up to two-thirds of its length. Its bark is relatively smooth, gray on the outside and red-brown on the inside. The wood is extremely hard (the "South American oak"), can take a great deal of mechanical strain, and has a lovely green-brown to green-yellow coloration. The sap vessels running through the wood contain yellow crystals, the so-called *lapachol*. The lapacho bears beautiful blossoms, 4 cm to 7.5 cm in length and 1 cm to 5 cm in diameter, from December to February of each year. These look a bit like trumpets, with a color that ranges from rose-pink to dark red on the outside and golden

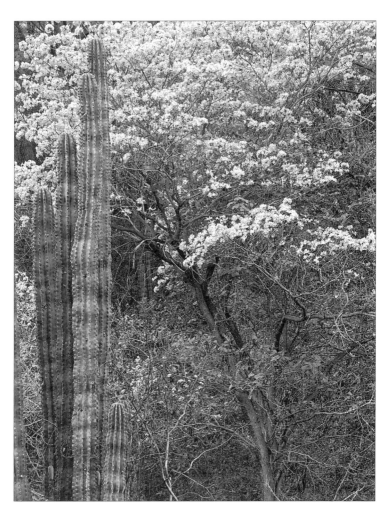

*A lapacho tree in full bloom growing wild in South America*

yellow to light yellow in the depths. You can find these beautiful flowers pictured on the cover of this book.

The lapacho tree has been cultivated for years as a timber in many places or grown on plantations for tea production. Despite the fact that the "divine tree" has been known in many areas of South America because of its extensive healing powers, there still haven't been any comparative pharmacological studies of all its manifestations (regional species) so that we don't even know to this date whether all lapacho species possess the same, or at least similar, active ingredients. However, there is much evidence in this direction, even if some representatives of the genus appear to be more effective for certain symptoms. The two modern "discoverers" of the healing power of pau d'arco, Professor Walter Accorsi and Dr. Theodoro Meyer, assess the tree with the purple-red flowers to be the bearer of the greatest medicinal powers. The major portion of the internationally marketed bark tea also originates from this variety.

Be that as it may: Indio tribes have been using the different species of this plant for similar purposes for centuries. Even the ancient Incas and Aztecs were already familiar with the tree's healing powers and liked to take advantage of its help. The shamans of the Amazon rainforest consider it to be one of the rare, truly great teacher plants, under special conditions capable of explaining the medicinal and spiritual uses of other plants to a person who is open for this.

For example, pau d'arco is offered in almost every pharmacy and herb store in the form of tea. Frequently, it is also on stock as homeopathic preparations. In the USA, hundreds of thousands of health-conscious Americans have already been using the tea and the capsules and extracts made from it since the end of the Eighties. The result has been extremely positive reports on experiences.

The species from which the medicinal drug (tea) is primarily produced for the world market is the *Tabebuia impetiginosa*, as well as the *Tabebuia avellandedae*. In contrast to this, almost all species of the lapacho are used as a strong, versatile healing remedy. However, not all species of the "divine tree" can be applied for health purposes as easily and free of risk for a person's health as the T. impetiginosa. Since, according to my knowledge, species with side effect aren't used to produce tea for the international supply, we don't need to worry when enjoying pau d'arco. For many years now, we have been able to purchase it in tea shops, natural food stores, pharmacies, and health food stores. Doctors and healing practitioners highly recommend it.

---

THE MANY NAMES OF THE DIVINE TREE

*Tabebuia impetiginosa* is also known in the scientific world under the following synonyms:

- Bignonia heptaphylla
- Gelseminum avellandedae
- Tabebuia avellanedae
- Tabebuia nicaraguensis
- Tecoma adenophylla
- Tabebuia dugandii
- Tabebuia heptaphylla
- Tabebuia ipe

---

INCLUDE SUCH TERMS AS:

- Acapro
- Alumbre
- Amapa (prieta)
- Bastard lignum vitae
- Bethabara
- Bow stick or bow tree[1]
- Canada
- Canaguate
- Caroba
- Chicala
- Coralibe
- Cortés
- Cortez
- Ebano verde
- Ebene vert
- Flor amarillo
- Groenhart
- Guayacan (polvillo)
- Hakia
- Ipe (roxo)[2]
- Ironwood[3]
- Lapacho
- Lapacho negro
- Madera negra
- Pau d'arco (roxo)[4]
- Polvillo
- Surinam greenheart
- Tabebuia
- Taheebo
- Tahua
- Tahuari
- Taji
- Tamura
- Verdecillo

*The correct botanical terms are:*
*Family:  Bignoniceae*
*Tribe:    Tecorneae*
*Genus:   Tabebuia Gomes ex DC.*

---

[1]  Bow stick since even the Incas liked to use it because of its outstanding mechanical properties as a material for carving highly resilient hunting and fighting bows.
[2]  "Ipe" is a Portuguese word for "bark" and "roxo" means "red."
[3]  Ironwood because of its great hardness
[4]  Bow stick or bow tree

I've compiled this list of synonyms because perception of one's own path in the cosmic context is offered and described under many different names. However, it's always intended to basically mean the same plant. At the beginning of my search, this was very confusing to me. If you would like to do some further research, this list will make it much easier for you. In terms of popular science and in the trade, the most frequently employed names are pau d'arco in the USA and Canada, lapacho in Europe, and ipe roxo and pau d'arco in the Portuguese-speaking countries.

Chapter 2

# The Discovery of the Lapacho Tree's Healing Power

The astounding healing power of lapacho bark first became known through the scientist Professor Dr. Walter Accorsi, MD and pharmacologist (University of Sao Paulo, Brazil), the botanist Dr. Theodoro Meyer, and the physician Dr. Pratz Ruiz in Argentina.

Since the beginning of his professional career as a botanist, Professor Accorsi dedicated his life to researching medicinal plants. Far beyond Brazil's borders, he was known for his vast knowledge of this field and also valued by colleagues from the medical world and the pharmaceutical industry as an expert.

While examining the lapacho tree's inner bark, he quickly came upon two essential, therapeutically useful qualities. On the one hand, it caused pain to disappear, and on the other hand, it brought about a distinct increase in the number of red blood cells, the task of which is to transport oxygen to the cells of the body. This means that the amount of red blood cells has essential significance for the recovery and regeneration processes of all types, as well as for the fundamental vitality of the organism. According to this perspective, pau d'arco has an effect similar to that of an oxygen treatment. Also compare this with "Chapter 3—This Is Why Pau d'Arco Is So Effective."

Convinced by a host of substantiated stories of healing from the population and reports from friends and colleagues, Professor Accorsi recommended pau d'arco for the treatment of various ailments, among which in particular were diabetes, cancer leukemia, ulcers, and rheumatism. As the experienced scientist emphasized to journalists of the popular magazine *O Cruzeiro*, his studies (at the end of the Sixties) hadn't yet met the standards of strict academic criteria.

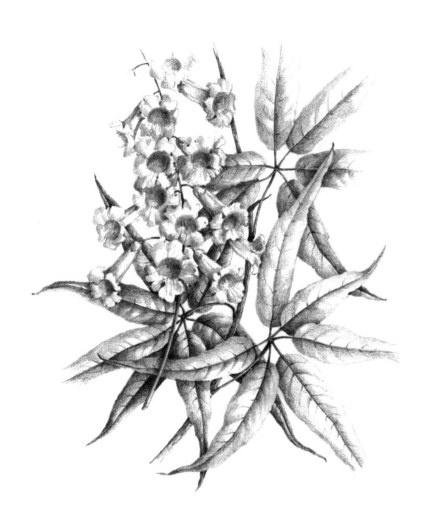

However, he would still stand up for his recommendations because there were simply too many positive reports of experiences and his studies of the components had also shown very good results.

*Important*: In the evaluation of the patient reports, it was conspicuous that distinct improvements of complaints, even for the most severe ailments, astonishingly occurred even after a few days or weeks!

Dr. Meyer of the state University of Tucuman in Argentina had already isolated the most important components of pau d'arco during the Sixties and discovered a quinone with a proved germicidal effect. Its structure is similar to that of vitamin K* and it has the following functions: a styptic effect through its support of the liver metabolism in the production of prothrombin and various substances that participate in blood coagulation. In addition, research results and reports on experiences indicate that it participates in the respiratory chain of the cell system and, as a result, improves the energy supply through the supply of oxygen to the cells. This leads to an understanding of why it should have a tumor-dissolving and anti-inflammatory effect because both health problems are accompanied by at least a partially diminished oxygen supply to the tissue. The vitamin-K complex within the human body is usually produced by healthy intestinal flora.** In addition, vitamin K occurs in all green plants to varying amounts. It is fat-soluble and heat destroys it, as in cooking.

Pau d'arco normalizes the composition of the blood. Used both internally and externally, it can, as shown in the example of millions of Indios for centuries, be a great help for a large variety of health disorders without fear of dangerous side-effects or interactions. To the contrary: The inner bark of the "divine tree" is even recommended in particular by

---

* Vitamin K (in more precise terms, there are a number of vitamins that work together. The two most important are K1, phylloquinone, and K2, menaquinone or farnoquinone.

** But who has completely healthy intestinal flora these days?!

doctors knowledgeable about herbs in order to ease or even prevent the problematic accompanying symptoms of chemotherapy, antibiotic treatments, and misuse of cortisone.

# A Scientist Learns from the Lords of the Medicine Bag

Dr. Theodoro Meyer, an Argentinean botanist who has received various awards for important research from the government, learned about the healing power of pau d'arco during his research visits to the Callawaya tribe. They are descendants of the Incas, and have probably produced the most famous plant healers of South America for the past millennium. Approximately one-thousand medicinal plants have been categorized by them and are also used today for treatment on a regular basis.* Like most traditional peoples in South America knowledgeable about medicine, the Callawaya also have prejudices against Western medicine and its representatives. It's completely normal for them to have one of their patients be treated by a physician with antibiotics and additionally give him or her a prescription for herbs. They also received Dr. Meyer with great openness and let him participate in their extensive traditional knowledge. This is where the great botanist learned much from the healers, who are respectfully called the "Lords of the Medicine Bag" by the

---

* Even at the beginning of the 20th century, the Callawaya healers already enjoyed a world-wide reputation as the "miracle doctors from the jungle." Their healing system was shown with great success at the Paris World Exhibition. During the construction of the Panama Canal, the Callawaya were called upon to treat the many workers suffering from yellow fever. The medicine of the Callawaya is based upon plant knowledge handed down from generation to generation, as well as being expanded and tested in practical terms time and again. This knowledge includes a diagnostic system and spiritual practices—like the mesa ritual—based in part on oracle and trance work. A Callawaya healer only begins a treatment if he has received a positive response when invoking his protecting spirits. For this reason, the healing rate of these "shamans of the Andes" reaches almost 100%.

people. Pau d'arco, they taught him, is one of the great "teacher plants." It can be used to heal and relieve a multitude of chronic health disorders and diseases, particularly cancer, leukemia, diabetes, and rheumatism. Fascinated by the "divine tree," he continued to do independent research and also maintained an active exchange of views with colleagues like Professor Dr. Walter Accorsi, who was also working on the topic.

For many years, the botanist worked at educating orthodox medical groups about the fantastic healing powers of pau d'arco—without success. He died, frustrated by the lack of understanding shown by established science, in 1972.

However, in recent years his research work on pau d'arco has been taken increasingly more seriously, as shown by the many clinical studies on the healing power of the "divine tree." However, the experiences of a growing multitude of enthusiastic pau d'arco users has long surpassed the slow recognition work of orthodox medicine.

## A Brazilian Professor Discovers Two Great Truths

In the year 1967, a newspaper interview with the physician Professor Walter Accorsi of the Municipal Hospital in Santa Andre, a suburb of Sao Paulo, caused a great deal of excitement. In this interview, the doctor explained that even in his initial experiments with pau d'arco it was possible to determine two remarkable effects: On the one hand, the tea quickly caused the disappearance of the frequently unbearable pain, which unspeakably torments so many cancer patients; on the other hand, the number of red blood cells were multiplied within a short time through the treatment with pau d'arco, thereby creating a much better supply of vital oxygen to the organism through the metabolism. He apparently recommended the tea for the treatment of many chronic ailments, which resulted in a lengthy period of time in which thousands of people lined up outside his practice seeking help. This situation was followed by animated discussions in the Brazilian media about the pros and cons of the pau d'arco therapy. Professor Accorsi distributed the bark of the "divine tree" to the sick for free and encouraged them to make a tea from it, as well as an alcohol extract, which was to be taken every three hours by the teaspoon. He didn't give any specific instructions on the dosage. In terms of this topic, he said tht there wasn't enough adequate data available on the active ingredients in pau d'arco. When the maximum of the daily amount to take had been reached by the respective person, he or she would experience a slight, completely harmless skin rash. The dosage should then be reduced somewhat. The skin manifestations would then disappear quickly and without causing any type of health problems.

However, the public announcement of the enormous healing power of the pau d'arco tea had negative aspects to it: Pau d'arco was never again prescribed—at least not officially—at the Hospital of Santo André since the prominent, large-scale reporting appeared in the magazine *O Cruzeiro*. The hospital management and many of the physicians were afraid of the ridicule and the international disparagement as quacks in their circle of colleagues. Previous to this time, pau d'arco tea and extracts from the bark had been used for years on a regular basis with greatest success at Santa André.

Yet, the world-wide, comprehensive scientific studies researching the healing power of the lapacho tree only began during the Eighties. Corresponding investigations were carried out in Japan, Germany, Scotland, Nigeria, and the USA, generally confirming the century-old experiences of the South American Indios without exception. However, one thing became increasingly clear: There wasn't just one individual "miracle active ingredient" in pau d'arco responsible for all the good results. Its extensive healing power originates in the totality of the substances contained within this plant, which we are completely justified in calling unique, and their fortunate balanced state and harmonious combination with each other. Becuase of the fantastic composition of the active ingredients, even the smallest amounts of the individual active ingredients can make a decisive contribution to processes like the inhibition of tumor growth. If the components are used in an isolated manner, much of their healing power disappears and the excellent tolerance and harmonious effect of the tea is often lost.

# Chapter 3

# Why Pau d'Arco Is So Effective

The healing power of the lapacho tree can't be traced back to one individual component. Only the unique combination of effective ingredients makes it broad therapeutic applications possible. In this chapter, I've compiled an overview of the components discovered up to now by scientific research, together with their significance. I ask the professionals among the readers to forgive me for portraying this information in a way that everyone can understand. An abundance of more detailed information for the various specialized areas can be found in the scientific publications listed in the appendix.

## Improvement of Oxygen Supply

There are large amounts of oxygen in the red inner bark of the lapacho tree, which is bound in a form easily available to the human organism and particularly valuable. Oxygen in this form can very efficiently kill bacteria, protozoa, fungi, and viruses. The body cells receive better nutrition—since oxygen can be termed their elixir of life—and coatings that impede the metabolism dissolve from the walls of the blood vessels. At the same time, the vitality and flexibility of these important blood vessels are substantially improved. The enzymatic activity* stimulated in the body on an extensive basis thorough the direct supply of oxygen. Furthermore,

---

\* Enzymes, called ferments in earlier times, are protein substances that facilitate and accelerate a variety of chemical reactions within the body in the role of catalysts, without changing themselves in the process. These are required for the transformation of the food in the intestines, as well as for fighting certain pathogens (germs) and maintaining the normal function of

pau d'arco promotes the formation of red blood cells to a high degree, thereby improving the possibilities for the transportation of oxygen within the organism.

These qualities of the "divine tree" were responsible for attracting the world-wide attention of researchers who were involved in the medical applications of oxygen. During the Eighties, a series of clinical studies resulted in clear indications that, for example, ozone injected intravenously or even the previously developed famous oxygen multiple-step therapy by Professor Ardenne can help the organism in many respects. With lapacho, a plant had been discovered for the first time that could be used as a source of oxygen, as well as for stimulating the formation of red blood cells in addition to other oxygen treatments. As a result, it's recommended that pau d'arco be used as a supplement for a great variety of ozone and oxygen therapies. In the same respect, the qualities of pau d'arco that have been mentioned here also make it quite useful for the improvement of wound-healing.

## Natural Antibiotic and Tumor-Healing Components

Lapacho bark contains various germ-killing substances. As early as the Sixties, the Argentinean botanist Dr. Theodoro Meyer discovered it to have a natural, holistically active antibiotic agent with negligible harmful side-effects (as long as it's used in connection with the entire biology of the plant). This substance, a quinone with the name of *lapachol*, was later also tested by the renowned *American National Cancer Institute* in terms of its healing power for tumors. Only in

---

the cell metabolism. Enzymes make an important contribution to the detoxification and purification of the body by transforming substances that are harmful or impede the metabolism and making them eliminable. For this reason, enzymes have also been increasingly employed in recent years in the therapy of chronic inflammations and for the treatment of cancer diseases. An ingenious pioneer of modern enzyme therapy was the physician Professor Max Wolf.

most recent times have more extensive tests been carried out in such countries as Germany, Scotland, Japan, and the USA. As a result, a total of twelve quinones with antibiotic qualities have been found.

However, the outstanding healing effects for which pau d'arco is so greatly valued result only in the complex interaction. These substances are also significant in relation to cancer diseases. They can inhibit the growth of tumors, kill cancer cells, and prevent the formation of metastases. Furthermore, when they occur together, only minor amounts are required for the comprehensive effect, including successful stimulation of the immune system!

*Bernhard Kreher*, a researcher from Munich, wrote his doctoral work on the immunostimulating effect of pau d'arco. He came up with these highly interesting results: The activity of the body's defense system was increased by more than 48%!

Moreover, pau d'arco contains a great deal of calcium and iron, which supports the transportation of oxygen, meaning the nourishment of the tissue and the immune system, and thereby strengthens the overall organism.

Selenium is contained in a comparably medium-strong concentration. Selenium is an important antioxidant, a catcher of the so-called "free radicals" that damage cells and cytoplasts, weaken the body's defenses, and promote the development of various diseases, or even trigger them—including cancer. Selenium may detoxify the body of the heavy metal *cadmium*, which is one of the most frequent environmental toxins today and causes high blood pressure and coronary diseases of the heart, among other things, as well as weakening the body's powers of resistance.

# Saponins Against Harmful Fungi and Cancer

The saponins, which are richly present in pau d'arco tea, are natural antimycotic agents that protect the body from harmful fungi and even create a climate capable of repelling them.

When herbal teas are given a powerful shake, saponins become visible in the form of foam.* When digested in the small intestine, the pau d'arco saponins facilitate the absorption of important active ingredients of other medicinal herbs that sometimes contain too little of these substances. This explains why herbalists of all traditions like to put pau d'arco tea into mixtures of various medicinal plants. According to experience, it intensifies the health-promoting effects of other components. In addition, some of the saponins contained in the pau d'arco tea are capable of reducing the growth of tumors. Japanese researchers, who discovered this characteristic, had a special pau d'arco saponin patented as a cancer drug for this reason.

# Pau d'Arco and Diabetes

In the traditional South American art of healing, pau d'arco is valued in the treatment of diabetes mellitus.

But what is the reason for this effect? The results of Brazilian research has been that pau d'arco inhibits the absorption of glucose (grape sugar) in the intestines. Because it quickly goes directly into the blood, without having to be further reconstructed by the metabolism, glucose increases the level of blood sugar in a way not tolerated by the organism. As a result, larger amounts of insulin are excreted by the pancreas in order to once again normalized the blood-sugar level. Often, the consequence of this is that hypogly-

---

* This also works with black tea—try it sometime!

The terms *diabetes* summarizes various forms of a disorder of the glucose metabolism. In diabetes it can always be observed that there is a relative or absolute deficiency of insulin, a hormone produced in the pancreas. This substance lowers the sugar content of the blood to a normal level that is beneficial to the organism. If too little insulin is produced, sugar crystals will deposit themselves on the walls of the blood vessels, for example, as a result of the level in the blood being too high. In diabetics, the overall metabolism is drastically disturbed by the organically non-utilizable excess of sugar. The susceptibility to infection increases, the vitality diminishes, defective vision develops, and the tissue on the arms and legs may die off due to the increasingly poor circulation. In terms of modern orthodox medicine, the treatment of diabetes generally occurs by having insulin supplied from the outside, maintaining a diet, and participating in motion therapy. Among other things, risk factors that promote the development of diabetes are: long-term high level of stress, a proportion of sugar in the diet that is too large, alcohol intake on a regular and excessive basis, chronic infections, and extreme overweight, as well as lack of exercise. Anyone taking an attentive look at this list won't have to wonder why this disease has been continually gaining ground in the Western industrial nations for years.

cemia occurs, triggering fatigue and an appetite for "something sweet." In industrial sugar is frequently eaten, either pure or "packaged," in larger amounts, the pancreas experiences such an extreme strain that it becomes damaged in its ability to produce insulin in cases of constitutional weakness or other negative accompanying circumstances (see box). If the absorption of glucose in the intestines is inhibited by pau d'arco, for example, this immediately relieves the pancreas. In addition, the metabolism is then caused to obtain its energy for the largest part from the utilization of long-chain carbohydrates. This supports the normalization of the appetite, the hunger decreases in some cases, and there is a growing tendency towards more healthy nutrition, as I have been able to ascertain from a series of reports on experiences.

In many cases, even within just a few weeks, provided no extreme nutritional errors are made, some of the overweight can be reduced in this manner without having to go hungry.

All of these are ideal preconditions for the pancreas to recover. Continue taking pau d'arco according to the instructions of Angelika Franz, MD for Naturopathy in Munich, which should have the effect of improving the function of the spleen-pancreas meridian. At the same time, pau d'arco:

- Exercises a healing influence on the delayed damage of diabetes by improving the supply of oxygen
- Prevents future metabolic problems
- Helps against tissue degeneration
- And, because of its antibiotic active ingredients that have no side-effects, helps heal inflammations (a great danger for diabetics and frequently the cause of limbs having to be amputated).

Because of these comprehensive health-promoting effects and its outstanding tolerability, pau d'arco should definitely receive a solid place in the therapy of diabetes. A person who can assume that he or she has an increased risk of diabetes* is well-advised to include pau d'arco as a house tea in his or her daily culinary fitness program.

---

* If diabetes has been manifested in parents or siblings, there is often an increased risk of a corresponding illness. If you would like more specific information and want to clarify your individual health situation with respect to diabetes, you should consult a physician who has been specially trained in the treatment of diabetes.

# Xyloidone: The Substance that Drives the Candida Fungi Out of the Body

An organic compound with the man xyloidone was identified by researchers just a few years ago as an important factor for the antimycotic (fungi-killing) effect of pau d'arco tea in relation to the candidiasis infections that have been occurring with increasing frequency. Xyloidone also possesses remarkable antibacterial and antiviral qualities.

# Lapachol—The Efficacy Carrier that Has Been Most Researched Up to Now

One of the quinones mentioned at the beginning of this chapter is called lapachol. It was already discovered during the Sixties by Dr. Theodoro Meyer, one of the two pioneers of modern pau d'arco research. He produced the first reports about the tumor-inhibiting and anti-inflammatory qualities of this substance. In the following decades, various scientists from around the world have researched lapachol extensively in laboratory tests and clinical studies. The following statements can be made about it today:

- Lapachol develops a distinct antiviral activity, among other things against: polio pathogens type 1, herpes simplex type 1 and 2, and various flu germs.
- The anti-inflammatory qualities of lapachol are considerably stronger than those of phenylbutayone, for example.
- Ulcers are healed by lapachol. The substance even prevents the development of gastric ulcers, which can be caused by excessive stress.
- Lapachol can frequently relieve pain caused by cancer diseases.
- Lapachol shouldn't be used in an isolated form during pregnancy.
- The very low concentrations of lapachol in tea, extracted from the inner bark of the tree, activate various immune

cells in the human body, the lymphocytes and the granulocytes. Considerably higher concentrations don't have such a good effect in this regard.

- ❧ Even malaria can be treated using lapachol.
- ❧ In an isolated form, meaning removed from the biological context of the original plant, and in high doses of 1500 mg and more a day, lapachol clearly diminishes the ability of the blood to coagulate and causes nausea and vomitting. According to Dr. J. B. Block, main author of the clinical studies on lapachol by the American National Cancer Institute, not even with these high doses can any type of toxicity be established with regard to the liver and kidneys. In the clinical applications, there have been successful tests in which the diminished blood coagulation caused by the lapachol was remedied by the additional administration of vitamin K. A distinct antitumor effect has resulted with the dosages stated above.

Unfortunately, time and again the effect of the pau d'arco bark tea has been equated in publications with the effect of lapachol. This is absolutely false. Although lapachol is a component that occurs in high concentrations in the heartwood, there are only trace of it in the bark. Lapachol in an isolated form is a remedy that is quite aggressive, even though there is no doubt about it being medicinally versatile. In its effects, the pau d'arco tea is very harmonious by comparison. Nature has brought together a concert of greatly varying healing substances in the bark of the lapacho tree. This successful synthesis alone distinguishes its uniqueness. It can in no way be limited to individual substances. To the contrary: If the natural context is lost, side-effects of all types occur, something that is sufficiently familiar from other isolated active ingredients.

# Further active ingredients

There is naturally an entire series of further important active ingredients in pau d'arco tea, such as veratric acid and veratric aldehyde, both substances that strongly stimulate the immune system in different ways, and further substances like various naphthoquinone derivatives, which demonstrate significant healing power. However, I have consciously refrained from describing these in detail here since knowledge of them is unnecessary for the practical use of the tea, and a certain amount of scientific knowledge is required to understand the immunological correlations. If you are interested in this topic, please consult the excellent work by Dr. Bernhard Kreher, listed in the appendix on page 120 "What's in pau d'arco tea?". Dr. Kreher has probably carried out the most comprehensive analysis of pau d'arco to date. Specialists will get their money's worth here. One important result of his work has been, among other things, that the optimal stimulation of the body's own immune system occurs through just tiny traces of the active ingredient in the pau d'arco tea.

# Chapter 4

# Does Pau d'Arco Tea Have Possible Side-Effects?

During my research, it was hard for me to believe that I couldn't find any warnings about the side-effects, interactions, overdoes, or counterindications against this medicinal plant anywhere.

Still, I did come across some information from the National Cancer Institute (USA). According to this, very high doses of lapachol, an isolated component of pau d'arco tea* can cause nausea, vomitting, and a diminished ability of the blood to coagulate.

This could naturally lead to uncertainty regarding the use of pau d'arco. For this reason, I would like to clearly state at this point: The dosages recommended in this book are generally in common use among those who give naturopathic treatments and have been used for many years without problems. It is also completely justifiable to recommend pau d'arco as a house tea, meaning a beverage to be consumed in larger amounts on a regular basis beyond the therapeutic applications, with prophylactic characteristics and a good taste to it. It has been used in this form for centuries by the Indios in large portions of South America and Central America. To the same extent, the reports on experiences by many users from Europe, Australia, Japan, the USA, and Canada are now available. These show the use of pau d'arco as a daily beverage in normal amounts, meaning—according to age, size, and weight—from 0.3 to 1.5 liters a day, to be not only quite safe but totally worth recommending.

Both the experienced botanist Dr. Theodoro Meyer and the physician Professor Walter Accorsi, who have intensively studied the applications of pau d'arco, agree that pau d'arco

---

* See information in previous chapter on this.

can be enjoyed quite safely by men, women, and children of all ages, and even by pregnant women. After years of research, the only sign of an extreme overdose that has been found is a moderate itching and a slight rash that disappears within a short time when the amounts given are reduced.

During the middle of the Eighties, tests with pau d'arco tea on laboratory mice were done at the University of Hawaii. These prove that it has no toxic effect. Even with a daily dose of 2 grams per kilogram of body weight, no type of organic damage could be observed in these experiments.

By way of contrast, pau d'arco tea rates much better in terms of toxicity than a beverage that is widespread throughout the world—coffee.* In plain English: If you find it easy to tolerate three to five cups of coffee per day, you can also be certain of having no problems with the same amount or more of pau d'arco. I won't even mention the other side-effects of coffee, which pau d'arco doesn't have.

If you would like to have two very simple rules as a basis for determining whether your body would like to have more pau d'arco or has had enough for the time being, then pay attention the following:

1. As long as you feel like having pau d'arco, it can be consumed without hesitation. But if an aversion to it arises, then reduce the amount for a period of time and drink something else in addition to it or instead of if. This could be catuaba or green tea, both of which also possess significant health-promoting characteristics. This "appetite rule" uses your own body signals as a gauge. Your body generally best knows its own need for certain foods.

2. As Dr. Theodoro Meyer discovered, the individual maximum dose can be determined quite simply in that when there is an overdose, a slight itching of the skin and a weak rash occurs. These manifestations quickly recede once

_____

* According to a study by the United States Department of Agriculture (USDA).

again as soon as the daily amount is reduced. The symptoms aren't serious and leave no problematic effects behind.

Some species of the lapacho tree contain greater amounts of tannin, a substance that also occurs in black tea and coffee. When beverages containing a considerable quantity of tannin are consumed in large amounts and frequently very hot, the mucous membranes in the cavity of the mouth and throat, the esophagus, and the stomach may become damaged. Although most of the pau d'arco teas available on the market are relatively low in tannins, you should still preferably drink the tea when it's lukewarm or cooled since even larger amounts won't have any problematic effects on the mucous membranes. Here is another solution: Tannins are bound by even just a few drops of milk or cream.

By the way, the recommendations in this section also apply to tea and coffee to the same extent!

**In concluding this chapter, here is one further bit of information:** There are a few species of the lapacho tree that bear white or yellow flowers, for which the good tolerance described above doesn't apply. Although these trees have traditionally had great healing powers attributed to them, the teas and tincture from their inner bark are only employed in very small amounts as medication with a high degree of efficacy. They aren't used as house teas because larger amounts of them can cause skin damage and trigger metabolic problems. The material composition of these lapacho species differs substantially in part from the varieties with purple-colored flowers. To my knowledge, the bark of the problematic representatives of this genus can't be found on the market.

SUMMARY

There aren't many semi-luxury foods that are as healing and tolerable—even when used over a longer period of time—as pau d'arco. However, when I write a book I consider it my responsibility to illuminate the topic from as many aspects as possible so that the reader can get a comprehensive overview and be able to evaluate possible risks.

# Chapter 5

# Enjoying Pau d'Arco Tea: Proper Preparation

What you must absolutely know before you make your first pau d'arco tea: In no case should you cook or store the tea in a pot containing aluminum or tin! These metals enter into a chemical compound with various components of pau d'arco tea when heated and therefore considerably reduce its medicinal effect. Other materials like glass, cast iron, ceramic, porcelain, steel, or clay are well-suited. Likewise, the tea shouldn't come into contact with plastic! Although it doesn't make it ineffective, a weakening of the effect may occur depending on the type and composition of the plastic. This also applies to the cut bark!

If you drink pau d'arco as a preventative treatment, meaning not as a health-maintaining house tea, it should be enjoyed unsweetened and between meals on an empty stomach.

The temperature should be lukewarm to cool. The requirement for one day is between three mugs of 0.2 liters and two liters, depending upon whether an intensive effect is desired or if a person has a very massive stature.

Since pau d'arco is a natural product, exact statements about the individual dosages can't be made. In addition, according to the reports on experiences that I have received, the exact dosage is less important for the effectivity than its use on a regular basis. The health-promoting components of pau d'arco are mainly represented in the small and smallest doses. According to many scientific studies, it has such a gentle and good effect precisely for this reason.

If you plan to drink it in larger quantities, you can prepare the appropriate amount for the entire day at one time. If you prefer to enjoy pau d'arco warm, you can cook it in the morning, fill it into a large thermos, and then take portions of it throughout the day. Please keep this in mind: When drinking larger portions of the tea, it shouldn't be any hotter than lukewarm. Pau d'arco can also be consumed cold.

# Basic Pau d'Arco Tea Recipes

For 6 mugs of 0.2 liters each (= 1.2 liters), put 1 to 2 slightly heaping teaspoons (about 5 to 10 grams) of pau d'arco tea, according to your taste preference, into the bubbly, boiling water. Then cover and let it simmer on a small flame for 5 minutes. Take the pot away from the heat and allow the tea to draw for about 15 – 20 minutes. Then pour the finished tea through a fine-meshed sieve or, even better, into a storage container through a linen cloth so that the fine pieces of bark are separated from the liquid. Otherwise, the drink will be slightly bitter.

I usually prepare two or three liters of tea at one time and keep a portion of it cooled. As a cool thirst-quencher, it tastes wonderful. There are some recipes for this on the following pages.

If you like it sweet, you can naturally add honey or raw sugar.

But please remember: If you desire a far-reaching, health-promoting effect, it shouldn't be sweetened!

The recipes described in this chapter have been put together in such a way that the good aroma makes sweetening unnecessary.

Here's a tip to fully develop the taste of pau d'arco: Don't keep the tea in the container in which it was prepared. Immediately after the cooking time is over, pour it through a close-meshed sieve or, even better, through a tea strainer made of cloth or a linen cloth into a pot. In this way, the little pieces of bark, which would otherwise remain in the tea and make it bitter and too strong, are held back.

On the other hand, I have heard from some pau d'arco connoisseurs that the strong aroma that develops when it draws for a longer period of time can be an interesting variation on the taste. The tea then has a spicy touch. Some South American Indio tribes basically don't remove the stock for the reason, particularly when the tea is used to promote digestion after a fatty, rich meal.

So just try it out. By the way—the strong preparation method tastes very interesting with rock candy and vanilla cream. It's worth a test in any case.

# Herbal Consecration— Mysterious Ritual of the Native Peoples

Perhaps you may have already heard that even in our overly civilized Western world some people who are very successful in working with medicinal plants* think that certain prayers spoken at the harvest and before using them can tremendously increase and intensify the medical effects of medicinal plants.

The fact is that the practice of herbal consecration or the blessing of herbs has been widespread since time immemorial. And rituals that have been used by many people throughout the generations must be based on a good reason. I have seen many reports on experiences and have had a

---

* For further information on this, please see the works of the medicinal-plant experts Wolf-Dieter Storl and Melli Uyldert listed in the Commented Bibliography of the appendix.

## A Shamanic Herbal Consecration For Increasing The Healing Powers Of Pau D'Arco

Look for a quiet place and have a supply package of pau d'arco, a candle, and matches ready.

**Step 1:** Hold the candle and say the words: "I hereby consecrate this light in my hands to the divine power and request healing."

**Step 2:** Take the bag with the pau d'arco tea between your hands and hold it at the level of your heart. Out loud or in your mind, thank the Earth Goddess who gives the plants their nutrition and support, and then the God of the Heavens who gives the sunlight, air, and rain that lets the plants thrive. Thank the spirits*, the four directions of the heavens, the forests, waters, and stones, and all other beings who have contributed to the growth of the healing plants that you now hold between your hands and have made sure that they could get to you. Thank the plants who have given you a part of themselves so that you will feel better.

**Step 3:** Say: "I request the healing blessing of the creative force for these plants. May their healing power fully awaken and give each person who enjoys them healing in the way right for him or her. (Only use the following section if you have an ailment that you would like to heal.) I ask to learn from my health disorder what is important so that I no longer need to suffer and can fully apply my strength for the realization of my new perceptions. I give thanks for the teaching."**

---

\* A collective term for spiritual beings, helpers of the creative force such as the angels or the Native American power animals.
\*\*The shamanic art of healing assumes that every disease contains an important message for the personal development of the person who is sick. If the afflicted person opens up to the lesson, a higher purpose will come into his or her life, making it easier for the individual to become healthy and developing more strength and maturity of character than before the illness.

**Step 4:** Wait a few minutes and feel what's going on inside yourself. Then give thanks and end the exercise by putting out the candle. The pau d'arco tea has now been "activated."

series of very convincing ones of my own that also speak in favor of this. So I would like to explain how you can also employ the herbal blessing yourself. You don't need to be a trained shaman or medicine man (woman) to do this. And for the skeptics: What do you have to lose if you just simply try this out a few times in order to examine the possible effects yourself? We all know that the proof of the pudding is in the eating!

# A Selection of the Best Pau d'Arco Recipes

### RECIPE 1—MINT PAU D'ARCO

When you put the tea in a cool place, add a twig of fresh mint or a slightly heaping teaspoon of dried mint to 1 to 1.5 liters. Although this is actually a recipe for cold tea, I know that it's also very delicious warm since I sometimes can't wait until it cools down.

### RECIPE 2—LEMON PAU D'ARCO

Add the juice of one to two whole lemons from organic cultivation, grate some of the peel into the tea, and decorate the mug with a few strips of it. It's best to sweeten this with raw sugar, apple herbage, or sugar-beet syrup.

### RECIPE 3—APPLE PAU D'ARCO

Add a good handful of dried apple pieces that have been cut down to size in advance to the tea (1 to 1.5 liters—according to taste) while it's still hot, together with a vanilla pod, and put it in a cool place. Don't drink it too cold. Because of the apple, the tea is already slightly sweetened, therefore it doesn't necessarily need additional sugar or the like, even for the tastes of someone with a sweet tooth. If you like, you can also vary this recipe by using cinnamon.

### RECIPE 4—THE COLD-KILLER, AN ALTERNATIVE TO GROG

Prepare the pau d'arco tea according to the basic recipe and then add 2 pinches of dried ginger root, a pinch of cayenne pepper, and the juice of an entire lemon from organic cultivation per liter of tea. This mixture will get your powers of resistance going within a short time and has a lasting effect if you drink it warm at the first signs of a cold. It causes most people to start sweating profusely. This is good for the elimination of toxins and waste materials, as well as activating the immune system. As a result of the slight temperature increase in sweating, the activity of the enzymes within the body is increased by more than 100 percent. The enzymes then provide a quick eradication of substances hindering the organism in its normal functions and also more easily put a stop to many pathogens. A fever may sometimes develop for a short time, which is a sign of how dynamically the organism has been activated against the illness.

### RECIPE 5—PAU D'ARCO A LA CREME, A SPECIALITY FOR SWEET TOOTHS (VARIATION I)

While the tea is still hot and drawing (see basic recipe), add an entire vanilla pod that has been squeezed out, together with a heaping tablespoon of candied orange and lemon peel from organic cultivation, as well as some cloves. Decorate with whipped cream topping before serving. This mixture not only tastes good but also has a slightly aphrodisiac effect!

### RECIPE 6—PAU D'ARCO A LA CREME; A SPECIALITY FOR SWEET TOOTHS (VARIATION II)

Prepare pau d'arco tea according to the basic recipe. Whip cream with genuine vanilla and some raw sugar. When serving, mix in one heaping teaspoon of whipped cream per mug and sprinkle with some cinnamon.

### RECIPE 7—FRUITY PAU D'ARCO

Prepare pau d'arco tea according to the basic recipe. When it has cooled down to drinking temperature, add one-quarter liter of cherry juice (from organic cultivation). This will preserve the valuable ingredients of the fruit juice. Tastes good warm and cold! If you like, you can also put a spot of whipped cream on top and decorate with grated almonds or other nuts.

### RECIPE 8—PAU D'ARCO FOR CHLDREN

According to my experience, children are particularly fond of pau d'arco tea as a cooled refreshment. It's also good to mix with apple or orange juice. When larger amounts are necessary because of an illness, shake the content of one pau d'arco capsule (also see Chapter 8, page 83 respectively into the milk bottle or the porridge and mix well.

### RECIPE 9—BRAZILIAN PAU D'ARCO

The following, quite unusual pau d'arco recipe comes from Brazil. A doctor living there invented it for his dying brother who was suffering from a cancer disease. The formulation is said to have been so effective that the patient, whom orthodox medicine had already given up on, was completely healed after one month.

Prepare the pau d'arco tea according to the basic recipe. However, use a dry white wine instead of water! After it has cooled down, fill with orange juice according how you want it to taste. To your health!

# Chapter 6

# Reports on Experiences and Pau d'Arco Stories

In this section of the book, I have compiled some anecdotes and stories about pau d'arco. They have been gleaned fro the international data highway in part, as well as from diverse publications on pau d'arco, and some have been told to me by the doctors I know.

## The Cancer-Afflicted Girl, the Monk, and Pau d'Arco

The Brazilian magazine *O'Cruzeiro* reported during the Sixties on the following case: A girl living in Rio de Janeiro had a sever cancer disease, and medical therapies didn't help her. She then began to pray urgently to God. She pleaded for help time and again, for something that could heal her. One day, she experienced an impressive vision in which a monk promised her that the tea from the inner bark of the lapacho tree would heal her. When she excitely told this to her parents, they didn't quite believe her. The father and mother were convinced that she had become psychologically unstable because of the serious illness, fleeing into fantasies out of disappointment in the unsuccessful medical treatments. Yet, the girl had one more vision in which the monk, apparently a spiritual guide, once more urgently advised her to take the treatment with the tea. Now the parents took the message seriously enough to permit her to try the remedy. The condition of the child improved increasingly afterwards, and she completely recovered after a few months!

## Cancer Tumor on the Scalp

An 86-year-old Brazilian suffered from a large tumor on the scalp. The physician treating him used topical compresses with pau d'arco tea and stock, which completely healed the severe illness without any further measures.  A follow-up examination of the man at the age of 92 resulted in no signs of cancer disease whatsoever.

## Constipation

A middle-aged American woman had suffered from stubborn constipation for years.  No matter what remedy she used—nothing helped.  It was so bad that she had difficulties going to work after a while.  When an acquaintance recommended the pau d'arco treatment to her, she reacted quite skeptically.  However, she did let herself become convinced to try out the tea at least once.  She prepared it in the morning and took it with her to work.  Whenever she was thirsty, she drank some of it.  After a few days, her digestion had completely normalized and she felt better than ever.

## Diabetes

A successful Peruvian businessman who frequently traveled to look after his diverse business branches always has a big bag of pau d'arco in each of his offices.  In gratitude for the healing of his diabetes, he made the vow that he would always have pau d'arco on hand in order to immediately be able to give the wonderful medicinal plant to, and recommend it to, anyone who needs it.

## Hay Fever

A bank employee living in northern Germany had been plagued by hay fever every spring for the past eight years.  A doctor who was a friend of his recommended that he do a four-week treatment with pau d'arco capsules by taking two of them three times a day, in addition to the pau d'arco tea on a regular basis.  The treatment was carried out in February.  Since that time, he has no longer had any occurrences of hay fever (observation period of three years).

# Leukemia

In July of 1967, five-year-old Marie was in treatment at the Conception Hospital in Sao Paulo because of leukemia. Despite the medical treatment, her blood count was becoming worse and worse until the doctors of the clinic finally declared her condition to be hopeless. The desperate parents asked the senior physician whether there wasn't anything else that could help their little daughter. The answer was disappointing: "Not in this hospital!" But as the parents were leaving, they were approached by another doctor who was familiar with the case. He advised them to go to the clinic of Dr. Pratz Ruiz, one of the most experienced representatives of the pau d'arco therapy, as quickly as possible. In Dr. Ruiz's clinic, Marie was immediately treated with pau d'arco tea. She received as much as she wanted to drink every day. Within just one month, her "hopelessly bad" blood values had already improved drastically. After a bit more than two months, in September, the happy parents were permitted to take their daughter home from the clinic. She was released with perfectly normal blood values and considered healed. Clinical details of the case were described extensively by Professor Burgstaller in his interesting book *La Vuelta a Los Vegetales*, Buenos Aires, 1968.

# Overweight

Doris, an entrepreneur in his mid-forties living in Dusseldorf, received the same devastating information regarding her overweight of almost 70 pounds from her attendant physicians time and again: Her metabolism was simply too lethargic, which is why she gained weight so easily and diets could only give her "relief" for a short time. A healing practitioner discovered that a longer period of treatment with antibiotics during her youth had probably led to the chronically insufficient function of her metabolism. She was therapied with various naturopathic methods after the orthodox physicians from whom she had requested advice didn't know how to help her anymore. Although the new therapies slowly put a brake on her weight gain, it could hardly be said that she was losing weight.  Not only was this a personal difficulty for Doris, but also a professional one since she managed a company that manufactured high-quality cosmetic products.  So it was naturally also important for her to have a good professional appearance.  However, this resolute woman didn't give up looking for a solution to her problems.  And so learned about pau d'arco tea from a friend who she met at a trade fair.  He said that he had become familiar with it in the USA as a comprehensive metabolic rehabilitator and learned to appreciate it as such.  He didn't know if this medicinal plant had ever been successfully used for a slimming treatment.  But since her overweight was based on a metabolic problem it would probably be worth a try, especially since the tea had proved itself to be completely harmless and tasted very good.  Doris let pau d'arco become her house tea.  She took it along with her on trips.  Already after a few weeks, she began to lose weight, although she didn't adhere to any kind of diet plan in particular.  Her appetite had simply been reduced and she felt more vital and full of the joys of life than she had for a long time.  Although she previously really had to pull herself together to visit friends after work or go out with her partner once in a while, she now very much looked forward to this and could even stay up longer occasionally without having her eyes fall shut at work the next day.  Her husband also noticed her astonishing change with great joy.  His wife was becoming more attractive and it was now possible to go out and do things with her.  After about two years, she had achieved her normal weight.  Almost one-and-a-half years have passed since then and she has maintained her figure without a problem.  She still likes to drink pau d'arco on a regular basis, but does so in smaller amounts.  She now usually has two to three cups a day.  It simply does her good, she says.

## Uterine Cancer

The following case was also reported by Dr. Pratz Ruiz: A woman who was seriously ill with uterine tumors lived on the sugar plantation La Corona.  She had such terrible pain that friends had to stop her from throwing herself in front of the train that regularly passed on the nearby railway. She was prescribed pau d'arco tea, which she drank in large quantities. After ten days, not only had the constant bleeding disappeared but her pain seemed to have vanished. After a thorough examination in which nothing more could be found, her attending physician declared her to be healed.

## Varicose Veins

In Argentina, there was a medically confirmed case of ulcerous varicose veins having existed for 20 years with a complete and lasting healing of all symptoms within just 16 weeks. The treatment was solely done using a pau d'arco ointment (pau d'arco extract mixed into a neutral ointment foundation).

# Chapter 7

# More Well-Being with Pau d'Arco Tea from A – Z

For many centuries, the Indios of broad regions of South American who live in harmony with nature have generally used pau d'arco for fortifying the immune system and fighting parasites within the body, against cancer and diabetes, and for comprehensive detoxification and purification. The scientific research and experiences of many doctors who work naturopathically around the world have shown that pau d'arco directly and indirectly contains substances that have an antibacterial, antiviral, and antimycotic effect. It generally exercises a healing effect on the entire body, thoroughly purifies the blood, and is capable of expelling many parasites. At the same time, it's important to know that pau d'arco not only has an effect directly against pathogens, toxins, and waste materials but, when used on a regular basis, also trains the body's abilities to substantially look after these functions itself in a much improved manner.

A flu infection, for example, can not only be healed wonderfully with pau d'arco—as a result, the body also develops greater powers of resistance against this type of illness.

In the following list, I have compiled a series of health disorders for which pau d'arco has proved to be effective up to now. In addition, some tips for therapy have been included with every point. Please understand that the following statements are not promises of healing or an exhortation that you should treat diseases requiring professional medical care on your own. Before using the specific remedy, discuss it extensively with your attending physician.

# AIDS

Take a few pau d'arco capsules several times a day and drink a larger amount of pau d'arco tea daily over a longer period of time. Unfortunately, more specific general instructions for dosage aren't possible in this case. A physician should determine the dose and the various means of application (see below) for an individual and respectively adapt it to the changes in the clinical picture. In this case, an experienced homeopath can also make use of homeopathic potencies of pau d'arco. However, these must be made by hand.

The pau d'arco treatment builds up the entire immune system. The secondary infections that frequently occur in those infected with HIV, such as those caused by fungi, are battled by its active ingredients. The body as a whole is strengthened and tumor cells are dissolved or their renewed growth is made more difficult.

Pau d'arco strengthens the inner organs. This is especially important because orthodox medicine's standard course of treatment, such as with the medication AZT, has serious side-effects on the liver. However, the effective ingredients of the lapacho plant have an especially beneficial effect on this organ in particular. When there is skin cancer, pau d'arco compresses and pau d'arco baths should definitely be employed as an additional measure.

It is also recommended that the patient drink catuaba tea every day. This medicinal plant lifts the mood, builds up the nervous strength, and, according to the clinical research results quoted in Chapter 10, has a beneficial effect on the AIDS therapy. In a certain sense, the cells are immunized against penetration by the AIDS virus. In addition, the catuaba tea has the effect of strengthening the stomach. This is significant because the standard medications, such as AZT, employed by orthodox medicine for AIDS therapy, greatly strain the stomach and can at times even cause intensive nausea. In many cases, catuaba tea can considerably diminish these side-effects that burden the body and the psyche.

Of course, the application and dosage of the two medicinal plants should be determined and monitored by a doctor trained in naturopathy. For this reason, do not treat yourself with it. Pau d'arco and catuaba aren't miracle cures against AIDS, but many reports on experiences and some scientific studies have given clear indications that the two medicinal plants can at least have a beneficial influence upon the course of this terrible disease.

## Alcohol Dependency and the Consequences of Alcohol Abuse

Drink pau d'Arco tea for a period of at least four to six months for detoxification and normalization of the metabolism. During the first three weeks, adults should drink up to 1.5 liters a day, followed by about .75 liters to one liter daily. Take a bath, adding three to four liters of pau d'arco tea prepared according to the basic recipe, one to three times a week. Bathe for about half-an-hour each time. Also see "Chapter 8—Applications for Pau d'Arco, The Pau d'Arco Bath."

In addition, ginkgo biloba, ginseng*, and ginger may be helpful. In severe cases, concentrated pau d'arco extract in capsule form can be used in place of pau d'arco tea. For the method of application and dosages in this case, please talk to the attending physician, healing practitioner, or pharmacist. The preparations from the plants mentioned can be obtained without a prescription. The organism is thoroughly cleansed and regenerated through the pau d'arco treatment. In the course of the treatment, a distinct aversion to injurious articles of consumption like alcohol and tobacco frequently occurs. Even a desire for sugar is often considerably reduced or disappears entirely because the sugar metabolism becomes normalized. Anyone who doesn't reach for these injurious articles of consumption for reasons of pure habit will remain healthy. Additional important help of a psychological nature can and should (!) be found from places like Alcoholics Anonymous, which have already given

---

* Don't use this if you have high blood pressure!

invaluable help to addicts.  There are also specially trained addiction therapists.

Withdrawal treatments in the narrower sense can't be carried out with pau d'arco tea.  But the "divine tree" normalizes and strongly purifies the metabolism, particularly the sugar utilization, and can therefore be very helpful in this, as in every other type of addiction therapy.

## Allergies of All Types

Enjoy up to 1.5 liters of pau d'arco tea as a course of treatment for four to six weeks.  In severe cases, pau d'arco capsules can be used additionally. One of these capsules contains the concentrated active ingredients of about one liter of tea.  According to individual needs, take one to two capsules two to four times a day.  Don't forget, above all when the symptoms tend to be serious, work out an exact therapy plan with the attending physician.

## Amalgam Extraction

Do a course of treatment with pau d'arco tea over a period of four months or longer, until it's no longer possible to determine any type of strain using suitable measuring methods like a pendulum, applied kinesiology, or bio-resonance. The therapy can be supplemented by taking a pau d'arco bath once or twice a week and one to three mouth rinses with pau d'arco tea every day.  In this type of application, take a small amount of the liquid—one to two tablespoons—into the mouth and suck it through the teeth as in the oil-sucking treatment.  In no case should you swallow the tea used for the mouth rinse!

## Anemia (Deficiency of the Blood)

Because of its characteristics of generally improving the blood, strongly promoting the production of red blood cells, as well as the considerable amount of iron that it contains and is easily utilized by the organism, pau d'arco is practically predestined for the treatment of anemia.  Anemia often results because of long-term nutritional errors such as in vegetarians who don't take care to get enough additional iron and vitamin B12. Another cause can be found in chronic inflammations that lead to iron deficiency and a worsening of the blood's vital functions. In the first case, the diet must naturally be adapted to the needs of the body. To clarify the second case, a doctor who works on a naturopathic basis should definitely carry out an examination of the so-called focal diseases. Pau d'arco contains an entire series of highly effective substances that are suitable for the therapy of inflammations. This is why it can also be used here for the healing of the causes.

## Arterial Sclerosis

Pau d'arco tea thoroughly detoxifies and purifies the body. Blood vessels that are clogged with deposits will be cleared out over time. In addition, pau d'arco can favorably influence the causes of arterial sclerosis such as diabetes, chronic inflammations, and metabolic problems of all types, both directly and indirectly. If you have parents suffering from arterial sclerosis but don't (yet) have any of the corresponding symptoms, it would be good for you to use pau d'arco as a house tea and do a course of treatment with the tea one to three times a year. Moreover, a nutritional specialist should make up an individual diet plan for you.

## Arthritis

Do a course of treatment with pau d'arco tea until the symptoms disappear. Afterwards, pau d'arco should be used as your house tea and a six-week tea-drinking treatment should be done two to four times a year. Also use pau d'arco wraps around the afflicted joints every day and take pau d'arco baths as required one to three times a week.

## Bleeding

Immediately take two to four pau d'arco capsules, at best on an empty stomach, or drink a larger amount of tea. If necessary, repeat this after several hours. For external bleeding, additionally make about one-quarter liter of strong pau d'arco tea (the double amount as in the basic recipe) and prepare a hot compress of sterile bandaging material with it. Then place it on the wound. Cover the compress with a cotton cloth. Pau d'arco has been used for centuries by the Indios of South America for internal and external wound therapy since it prevents infections and improves the healing of wounds. Always make the tea fresh for wound treatment! If larger blood vessels are injured, a doctor must definitely be called as quickly as possible and first-aid measures must be taken in order to stop the bleeding. Even when small blood vessels are injured, the following applies: if the bleeding doesn't stop within fifteen minutes despite the pau d'arco treatment and correct first-aid measures, a doctor must be called to decide upon the further course of treatment. It may be, for example, that in addition to the bleeding there is also a blood-pressure level that is much too high, which is why the bleeding can't be stopped by normal blood ligation.

## Blood Improvement

Pau d'arco tea is excellently suitable for improving the vital characteristics of the blood and normalizing the overall blood picture since it thoroughly purifies the organism and has a beneficial influence on inflammations. Carry out the pau d'arco tea-drinking treatment until the values have normalized and the subjective complaints have disappeared.

The tea of the "divine tree" can naturally also be wonderfully employed within the scope of a springtime course of treatment for the general removal of waste materials.

## Bronchitis

Drink pau d'arco tea until complete healing has occurred, also inhaling the stream from hot pau d'arco tea under a towel several times a day. If there is a strong susceptibility to infection in relation to colds, use pau d'arco as a long-term house tea and do a pau d'arco course of treatment three to four times a year.

# Cancer, All Types

Take several pau d'arco capsules a number of times a day until healing has occurred. In addition, drink the tea as a course of treatment in accordance with your appetite for it. For skin cancer, the external application in the form of baths and compresses can also be recommended. Pau d'arco can be very useful when radiation or chemotherapy is employed. In some cases, these hard therapies can't be avoided. However, pau d'arco can often be used to harmonize the sometimes vehement side-effects of these types of therapy. The liver, intestinal flora, kidneys, and the entire body's own defense system are strengthened by the South American medicinal plant and can then better survive the treatments of orthodox medicine. According to reports on experiences, frequently the intense pain that occurs in many types of cancers is effectively reduced or even caused to disappear by pau d'arco.

In addition, catuaba can be used since it has the effect of a gastric tonic and mood-brightener. Particularly when there are longer-term radiation treatments and chemotherapies, this characteristic is worth its weight in gold.

It's important to treat cancer diseases as early as possible. For this reason, it's recommended that the individuals make use of preventative medical check-ups. Although these may only detect cancer diseases after they have reached a certain size, in most cases this is still long before there are distinct symptoms noticed by the person afflicted. Various naturopathic methods of diagnosis are appropriate for already showing the predisposition of a cancer disease (precancerous) even before it can be clinically determined. There are almost always typical metabolic derailments even many years before the occurrence of the disease manifestations that can be diagnosed by orthodox medicine. When a naturopathic therapy is used to normalize the overall metabolism during this generally complaint-free area, most operations, radiation treatments, and chemotherapies can be avoided. Tumors don't even occur at all. This is certainly the most elegant and safest type of cancer therapy according to the motto: "Prevention is better than healing!" The layperson can also take certain steps in order to discover a possible cancer disease in due time.

The seven signs that *could* be an early warning of cancer are:

1. Thickenings or knots form in the breast or other places in the body.
2. Changes in moles or warts become visible.
3. Are there lasting, clear changes in urination or defecation? Is this accompanied by pain? Can blood be seen in the excretions? Must the toilet be visited considerably more often or at much larger intervals of time than otherwise?
4. Continuing problems occur when swallowing or in digestion.
5. Discharge and bleeding of an unusual sort.
6. Hoarseness and coughing that just doesn't go away.
7. Wounds need longer to heal than otherwise, easily become inflamed again, or sore places remain.

**Please** don't drive yourself crazy if you discover some of these described symptoms in yourself. In addition to cancer, there are a great many other harmless reasons for them. Have yourself thoroughly examined by a doctor who uses holistic methods. Then you will have an exact idea of the situation.

Especially in the treatment of metabolic derailments, pau d'arco can be a wonderful help and is therefore, according to the information I have, excellent for use in *precancerous therapy*. During the treatment of cancer diseases of any type, sugar and white flour should generally be eliminated from the diet. They "feed" the cancer cells. In contrast to orthodox medicine, naturopathy doesn't structure the cancer therapy according to the symptoms alone but also assumes that:

1. The tumor cells must be destroyed.
2. The body's own immune system must be comprehensively built up and lastingly kept capable of functioning on a high level.

3. The environment within the organism must be changed in the direction of "health." In order to do this, toxins and waste materials are extracted and the living circumstances changed in such a way that a renewed blocking of the metabolism through an improper diet, for example, can be counteracted.
4. The psyche must be harmonized and oriented towards a primarily joyful life filled with meaning and love, taking responsibility for itself. (Also see my tips for mental training to this effect in the last chapter!)

Pau d'arco tea can directly cover the first three points and thereby effectively support any type of cancer therapy.

Although it's possible to support the fourth point through medication, it can't be decisively changed in this way. Only the affected person comprehending how to harmonize his or her way of life and inner attitude, as well as consequentially turning this decision into action, can provide help here for a positive, fulfilled life in the long term. Catuaba can also be helpful for this topic.

## Candidasis

Pau d'arco tea develops a strong, direct healing effect against some types of fungi that can do a large amount of damage to the human body—however, as many laboratory experiments have clearly proved, the tea of the lapacho plant is *ineffective* in the *direct* application against candida fungi. "Too bad," you are probably certain to think. But don't worry—the whole time this has just referred to the *direct* application. Pau d'arco has been very successfully used in South America for centuries against candida diseases. In the USA and Canada as well, there are hundreds of thousands of very positive reports on experiences with reference to the therapy of the insidious fungus diseases using pau d'arco. "How is this possible?," you may ask. Well, pau d'arco makes sure that the entire body is thoroughly detoxified and purified, which means that the immune system functions much better as a result. Some of its components have such an effect on the defense system that the production of immune cells, which attack the fungus spores, is drastically increased. In addition, the sugar metabolism is normalized. A derailed sugar metabolism is an invitation for candida! In addition, the liver, kidneys, and spleen are strengthened, and pau d'arco provides a considerably improved supply of oxygen to the body. Fungi don't like this at all.

According to my information, pau d'arco tea is one of the most effective healing remedies that we have against candida and other fungus diseases. Try it!

## Chemicals, Hypersensitivity to

In recent years, there have been increasingly more people throughout the world who already suffer in response to minor amounts of chemicals in a great variety of ways. They experience the symptoms of allergies, fatigue, a vague feeling of not being well, and other things. It should be noted: we aren't talking about poisoning through chemicals here! This deals with substances and amounts that are in no way conspicuous to people who aren't this sensitive. *Chemical hypersensitivity* has been successfully treated with pau d'arco in the USA. Tea-drinking treatments on a regular basis promise the best results here. As usual, this effect can be intensified by taking pau d'arco capsules.

## Colds

At the first sign of a cold, pau d'arco should already be put to use. For four days in a row, drink either 1 to 1.5 liters of pau d'arco tea or obtain pau d'arco capsules, which contain an extract of the bark, at the pharmacy. The effect of one capsule corresponds to that of one liter of tea! Application: take two capsules the first day and then again two capsules six hours later. Repeat this treatment for three days. This will so strengthen the immune system in a natural way that the cold can't even get a foothold in the organism. The nice thing is that pau d'arco not only improves the defense functions but also trains its ability to deal with each respective pathogen! But be careful: if you don't make it through three days of the pau d'arco flu treatment, the cold comes back again in many cases; even if it already appeared to be cured!

So don't become foolish because of the quick success. Drinking a great deal of liquids is also useful in this situation.

In addition, a flu bath can be prepared with the pau d'arco. Simply add about three liters of tea to the bath water each time and bathe in it for about 30 minutes every day until the end of the flu treatment.

By the way: The more you treat yourself naturopathically, the less often you will get a cold! Among other things, colds are a type of emergency purification for the plagued metabolism.

## Colitis, Ulcerative

Do a long-term tea-drinking treatment with pau d'arco tea, in addition to pau d'arco capsules and enemas with the tea. You must absolutely work out the details of the therapy with the responsible physician before doing anything. Have him or her constantly monitor the course of the treatment!

## Cystitis

Do a course of treatment with pau d'arco tea. Drink larger amounts so that the urinary passages are constantly being rinsed! Place pau d'arco compresses on a generously large area surrounding the bladder.

## Diabetes

Do a long-term tea-drinking treatment with pau d'arco tea, and definitely continue beyond the disappearance of the symptoms. Have a pau d'arco bath one or two times a week. According to the intensity of the symptoms, pau d'arco capsules can also be used during the first months. Before beginning the treatment with pau d'arco, you must absolutely inform the responsible physician since the frequently very quick normalization of the metabolism must be followed by a continual adjustment of the insulin administered. In no case should you do this on your own since serious consequences could occur without professional help!

If delayed damage such as serious circulation disorders, inflammations, and the like are already evident, pau d'arco should also be intensively used externally.

According to many reports on experiences from Brazil, the use of pau d'arco is also worthwhile for juvenile-onset diabetes!

## Discharge, Vaginal

Do a six-week pau d'arco tea-drinking treatment and daily vaginal douches with body-temperature tea. In addition, or in place of this, you can also use tampons that have been soaked in pau d'arco tea. Change the tampons two to three times a day. Discharge can also be caused by fungus infections, chronic inflammations, or parasites. The basis of these problems is a derailed metabolism in the entire body. This is why pau d'arco should always be used internally on a long-term basis as well. Also helpful for a direct healing influence on the metabolism in the pelvic region are warm pau d'arco compresses, which should be placed alternatingly on large areas of the abdomen and sacrum. If candida fungi are the cause of the symptoms, the local application can only bring a secondary benefit since the emphasis should be on the pau d'arco tea-drinking treatment here. For other types of fungi, the local application can often, as shown in reports on experiences, cure the symptoms within a few hours.

## Eczema

Treat as described under chronic suppurations. Eczema indicates a strong creation of metabolic waste products, chronic disorders of the digestion, and inadequate functioning of the liver, kidneys, and spleen.

## Eyelids, Paralysis of the

Do tea-drinking treatments with pau d'arco tea, as well as compresses on and around the eyes. Clarify the psychological causes.

# Eyes—Tired, Inflammed, or Irritated

If you work a great deal at a computer monitor, you will be familiar with this: irritated, strained eyes that itch and burn long after the work is done. Compresses such as cotton pads moistened with pau d'arco tea and placed on the eyes for 5 to 10 minutes can often work true wonders. Small glasses for eye rinses are also available in pharmacies and medical supply stores.

*A tip:* There are antireflective and grounded monitor filters from various manufacturers at affordable prices in specialty stores. If you work at a monitor on a regular basis, you should allow yourself to have something like this*. In addition, if you are highly sensitive in relation to the subtle disruptive fields, you can use electromagnetic-field reducing devices for your monitor.

## Facial Cancer

Use compresses with strong pau d'arco tea or the pau d'arco tea-drinking treatment. Otherwise, look under the key word "Cancer."

## Fistula

Do a tea-drinking treatment with pau d'arco tea, possibly intensified by pau d'arco capsules and topical applications until healing occurs.

## Fungal Infections (Mycosis)

For fungal diseases on the hands and feet:
Bathe the afflicted limbs twice daily for 15 minutes in a pau d'arco tea infusion for ten days. Prepare the infusion at twice the strength stated in the basic recipe. As a result, the fungi will be killed directly and the metabolism at the infected parts of the body considerably improved. During the time of the external application, drink the pau d'arco tea prepared according to the basic recipe in amounts of up to two liters a day. If the fungal infection is chronic, meaning that it has

---

* It's important to do nice things for yourself!

existed for several months or even years, a longer-term pau d'arco tea-drinking treatment should be done. To do this, drink up to 2 liters of pau d'arco tea, prepared according to the basic recipe, every day for six weeks in order to make the environment in the body intolerable for the fungi. For infants and small children, the tea can be added to the bath water and given in amounts up to about 500 ml a day as a beverage. For children up to 12 years of age, a liter of pau d'arco is usually adequate. For older children, give the full amount of one-and-a-half to two liters a day.

Fungi in the body are basically fought by a long-term tea-drinking treatment with pau d'arco. In addition, use pau d'arco capsules daily and a pau d'arco bath once a week. Instead of seasoning your food with black pepper, use cayenne pepper. If you like, you can also put a small (!) pinch of it in your pau d'arco tea now and then. Cayenne pepper is another powerful healing remedy against any type of fungus disease. However, it should again be emphasized that only small amounts are to be used. It's effective when taken on a regular and long-term basis. Furthermore, garlic can help in the healing of mycosis (fungus infections). In order to take advantage of its full active powers, it should always be carefully crushed before using it. This produces specific compounds of its ingredients, which have a therapeutic benefit.

Please heed: During a pau d'arco treatment for the healing of an inner fungus infection, it has frequently been observed that a worsening of the subjective and objective symptoms may occur for some time! The reason for this is the massive dying of fungi within the body, the related release of toxic substances, and the resulting burden on the metabolism. Yet, the more the elimination of the fungal toxins progresses, the more intensively the general condition improves. This naturally also includes the specific symptoms.

## Gastritis

Drink larger quantities of pau d'arco tea. In severe cases, you can also supplement the therapy by taking pau d'arco capsules at an interval of two to three hours.

## Granuloma Annulare

Do a course of treatment as explained under the key word "Fungal Infections."

## Hodgkin's Disease (Lymphogranulomatosis)

Inner application with a great deal of tea and supplementary capsules. Important: take pau d'arco baths on a regular basis and use a pau d'arco wrap on the affected lymph nodes every day.

## Inflammations

Use the course of treatment described under the key word "Suppuration."

## Joint Inflammation

Apply compresses with pau d'arco tea. Drink the tea in larger quantities for several days. For chronic joint inflammation, see under the key word "Arthritis."

## Kidney Inflammation (Nephritis)

Drink larger quantities of pau d'arco tea until the inflammation has healed. An extensive supply of liquids has a positive effect on infections of the kidneys and uretic organs. This is why tea is preferred over other applications here. In severe cases, capsules can naturally be used as a supplement.

## Leukemia (Cancer of the Blood)

Begin with the pau d'arco treatment as early as possible, at best with tea and capsules. Otherwise, see under "Cancer."

## Liver Disorders of Various Types

Since pau d'arco generally supports detoxification and purification, as well as fighting infections and fungi within the body, it's very well suited for relieving the liver metabolism and regenerating this organ. According to the doctor's recommendations, use pau d'arco capsules or tea until the disorder has healed.

## Lupus

Do the tea-drinking treatment with pau d'arco, supplemented by pau d'arco capsules. For external use, put pau d'arco compresses on the afflicted areas. If cortisone has been employed for therapy purposes over a longer period of time, the pau d'arco capsules should be used on a long-term basis.

## Mouth, All Types of Diseases

If there are health problems in the area of the mouth and throat, you can gargle and rinse with pau d'arco tea. Don't swallow the tea in this case.

## Multiple Sclerosis

Because of its anti-inflammatory and metabolism-normalizing action, pau d'arco tea has a beneficial effect on this disease, which is otherwise difficult to treat. Use long-term pau d'arco treatments, pau d'arco as a house tea and also in capsule form. A pau d'arco bath is recommended once or twice a week.

## Nose, All Types of Diseases of the

After inhaling the steam of the pau d'arco tea, the body-temperature liquid can also be drawn into the nose and blown out again a number of times.

## Osteomyelitis

Do a tea-drinking treatment with pau d'arco until the problem has healed. Definitely use pau d'arco capsules as a supplement and place wraps with strong pau d'arco tea on the afflicted areas of the body every day.

## Pain Conditions of All Types

Place pau d'arco compresses on the painful areas.

## Paralysis of the Eyelids

Do tea-drinking treatments with pau d'arco tea, as well as compresses on and around the eyes. Clarify the psychological causes.

## Parasitic Disease in General

For external infestation: Wash with strong pau d'arco tea and do pau d'arco partial or full baths. In very difficult cases, additionally brush pau d'arco tincture onto the afflicted areas of the body several times a day. Also drink pau d'arco tea over a longer period of time in order to improve the metabolism. Parasitic disease always means an intensive *accumulation of waste material* within the organism. This can be eliminated by pau d'arco, if used for an adequate period of time.

For internal infestation: Do a tea-drinking treatment with pau d'arco. Possibly supplement with pau d'arco capsules.

(Also see under the key word "Fungal Infections.")

## Parkinson's Disease

Do a long-term tea-drinking treatment with pau d'arco, supplemented by pau d'arco capsules and a bath with pau d'arco once a week.

## Polyps

Until the hypertrophy of the mucous membrane has healed, carry out a pau d'arco tea-drinking treatment. Intensify the effects during the first four weeks by taking the pau d'arco capsules. Additionally inhale the steam of pau d'arco tea under a towel two to three times a week.

## Prostatic Infection

Do a longer course of treatment with pau d'arco. Also chew pumpkin seeds. These contain active ingredients that have a beneficial effect on prostatic complaints. Apply pau d'arco compresses on large areas of the abdomen daily. Furthermore, there is a food supplement made from a certain type of cactus with the name *Opuntia* that is very effective in relation to infections of the prostrate gland. Drink large quantities—from 1.5 to 2 liters of liquids a day.

## Psoriasis

Do a tea-drinking treatment with pau d'arco until cured. In serious cases, supplement with pau d'arco capsules. Take whole-body or partial baths with pau d'arco in order to calm the afflicted areas of the skin and promote healing. In severe cases, additionally dab the afflicted parts of the body with pau d'arco tincture and apply pau d'arco compresses.

## Rheumatism

Do the pau d'arco tea-drinking treatment on a long-term basis and apply compresses to the painful areas. The treatment should be supplemented by pau d'arco capsules and pau d'arco baths on a regular basis.

## Ruptures (such as Hernia)

To accelerate healing, carry out a tea-drinking treatment with pau d'arco tea and apply wraps with pau d'arco stock to the afflicted areas of the body every day.

## Smoker's Cough

For purification of the metabolism, do a tea-drinking treatment with pau d'arco on a longer-term basis. Inhale the steam of pau d'arco tea under a towel once a day. Apply pau d'arco compresses to a large area of the chest several times a week. Take a pau d'arco bath once a week.

## Sore Spots on the Skin

Moisten the affected areas with pau d'arco tincture and bandage or apply compresses that have been soaked in strong pau d'arco tea. If the sore spots on the skin didn't occur because of injuries, at least six weeks of the tea-drinking treatment should definitely be done in order to adjust and detoxify the metabolism. An examination by a doctor who employs holistic methods is absolutely recommended. Also see under the key word "Cancer."

## Splenic Infections

Drink pau d'arco tea over a longer period of time or additionally take pau d'arco in capsule form in severe cases. Apply pau d'arco compresses to the spleen area.

## Suppuration

For chronic suppuration, do a six-week tea-drinking treatment with pau d'arco, supplemented with pau d'arco capsules in severe cases. Topically apply pau d'arco compresses. In addition, take full or partial baths with pau d'arco several times a week, according to the type and extent of the disease. If it's an acute occurrence, the emphasis should be on the local treatment and drinking larger quantities of pau d'arco tea until the healing is complete. In very acute cases, pau d'arco capsules should additionally be taken because of their stronger effects. For furunculosis, pau d'arco baths should be taken several times a week as well.

## Tobacco Withdrawal

(Also see "Alcohol Dependency" and "Smoker's Cough")
Do a long-term tea-drinking treatment with pau d'arco. If you have smoker's cough, inhale the steam of the tea under a towel on a regular basis. Additionally use the pau d'arco capsules.

## Ulcers of All Types

Treat according to description given under the key word "Suppuration."

## Varicose Veins

Do wraps with pau d'arco tea, particularly for acute complaints. Do the six-week tea-drinking treatment several times a year.

## Warts

In addition to a six-week pau d'arco tea-drinking treatment for the cleansing of the organism from waste materials and toxins, the warts can be brushed with pau d'arco tincture (available in the pharmacy or by mail-order) or treated with pau d'arco compresses several times a day.

## Wounds

Apply compresses with *freshly prepared* tea. Remember that the bandage should be sterile. For larger injuries, always use pau d'arco internally as well.

# Basic Information on Successfully Using Pau d'Arco

Be sure to *always* use pau d'arco on a treatment basis for a period of time after the respective symptoms have disappeared in order to avoid recurrences. pau d'arco then additionally builds up the organism's powers of resistance. But this requires a bit of time. For acute health problems, several days are usually completely adequate. But a bit longer with pau d'arco certainly can't hurt. For chronic diseases like cancer, multiple sclerosis, and the like, if they haven't progressed very far, you should follow the old naturopathic healing rule that says: "Per year of illness calculate about four weeks of healing time!" According to the perceptions of naturopathy, for example, a cancer disease begins about 10 years before the first clinically diagnosable symptoms can be proved.

In severe cases of so-called "incurable diseases" like leukemia, the afflicted person shouldn't stop with the pau d'arco treatment when the symptoms that can be clinically determined have subsided. Dr. Theodoro Meyer, one of the greatest modern authorities on the healing power of the "divine tree," recommended that pau d'arco be used for the rest of a person's life in such cases. The reason for this is that in advanced cases, the organism has often completely or partially lost its ability to lastingly keep itself in a healthy condition.

The diseases and pau d'arco applications listed in this chapter should naturally only be considered to be examples. Pau d'arco is suitable as at least a supportive therapy for almost every health problem, yet laypeople shouldn't act on their own but trust in the advice of an experienced, holistically oriented doctor.

I ask the professionals among the readers to forgive me for naming some of the applications a number of times, such as "Inflammations" and "Joint Inflammations." Since I think, and hope, that this book will be read by many laypeople, I have repeated certain applications that have been generally listed again in their special forms of manifestation.

# Chapter 8

# Applications for Pau d'Arco

## Pau d'Arco Tea

In my opinion, this is the most important and versatile form of administration. Through the type of preparation and the large amounts of liquid that reach the inside of the body in this manner, its detoxification and purification wonderfully supported. *Water is unconditionally necessary* in order to wash substances out of the body that aren't beneficial for it. In the other forms of administration, this essential basic rule is all too easily ignored. Moreover, in the process of preparing the tea, precisely the proper substances that to trigger an optimal and harmonious effect are dissolved from the bark. Corresponding academic studies have also proved the effects of tea as a form of preparation, although it scientifically still hasn't truly been explained why the tea, with its curative substances that sometimes just appear in traces amounts, can do such great things. This fact reminds me of homeopathy, where similarly minor doses can initiate intensive health-promoting processes.

## Pau d'Arco Capsules

On the one hand, this form of administration is recommended for intensive pau d'arco treatments involving serious diseases because a person can only ingest a limited amount of liquid. This naturally also sets an upper limit for the amount of the active ingredients that enter into the body.

On the other hand, pau d'arco capsules are precisely the right choice when you travel a great deal or can't spare the time to prepare and enjoy the tea on a regular basis for other reasons, but still don't want to do without the beneficial pau d'arco effects. But please remember: if you want to thoroughly eliminate waste materials and detoxify, the body will definitely need an adequate supply of liquid. The appropriate amounts vary between one-and-a-half and more than two liters for adults. Coffee, black tea, milk, sodas containing caffeine, and alcoholic beverages don't count!

If you want to *quickly* prepare a pau d'arco wrap, the capsules are very useful as well. Simply open two to four of them and sprinkle the powder on a compress moistened with hot water. Apply to the corresponding area of the body, wrap up with a cotton or wool cloth, and it's ready. However, the wrap made with freshly cooked pau d'arco tea is clearly superior in its effects. This is a type of "emergency recipe."

If you want to supply your pets such as dogs and cats with pau d'arco, to get rid of pests in the fur, for example, you an also have the four-legged pals drink pau d'arco tea. Many of them like it. However, you can also sprinkle the contents of a capsule into the meals, which makes times tough for the fleas and ticks.

## Pau d'Arco Tincture

This preparation is an extract on an alcohol basis (such as honey wine). The tincture is well-suited for travelling, but can also provide quick help for small injuries. Simply put some of the tincture on the wound—it will burn a bit because of the alcohol—and carefully bandage it. Drink the rest of the bottle in order to accelerate healing the wound from within. Compresses can also be made with the tincture if there is no tea and no hot water on hand when away from home.

## Pau d'Arco Compresses

This type of application is particularly suited for skin problems of all types, including the treatment of inflammations of the joints, tendons, and muscles, as well as for wounds of all types.

Prepare the pau d'arco tea twice as strong as described in the basic recipe, soak a cotton cloth in it, and place it on the appropriate area of the body. This cloth should naturally be clean and must absolutely be sterile (!) if the wound is open. The compress should be hot but obviously not so that it hurts or you even scald yourself! Wrap a second cloth made of cotton or sheep's wool and keep it in place with clamps or bandages. Be careful! The wrap should in no way cut off the supply of blood.

When the wrap has cooled down, it can be removed. Use it one to three times a day in fresh tea until the wound has healed. In severe cases, do this more frequently as required. For open wounds, a new, sterile cloth must be used each time and soaked in freshly prepared tea. The tea must also be sterilized! Consult a doctor on how to do this. In no case should you brew the old tea a second time. Germs could otherwise get into the injury. When using them for an open wound, the cloths must be boiled afterwards to ensure thorough cleaning.

Instead of the extra strong tea preparation, you can also simply use the stock that remains after you have cooked the pau d'arco tea according to the basic recipe. Take the stock when it's still hot, wrap it into a thin cotton cloth and apply it like a compress. As in the first case, wrap an additional cloth around it and fasten it in place.

## The Pau d'Arco Bath

Particularly for external diseases, pau d'arco baths can be a very effective application. So that an optimal effect occurs, please pay attention to the following:

Prepare about one-and-a-half liters of tea according to the basic recipe but twice as strong as described there. Pour the finished tea into the bathtub, which should be filled with bath water at slightly more than body temperature (about 38 to 39 degrees Celsius). Caution! Don't use any further bath additives! Bathe for about half-an-hour without soaping down or washing your hair. (You can do this beforehand.) Afterwards, don't shower or rinse the skin. Just dry it lightly. Wrap yourself up in a pre-warmed fleecy bathrobe or a large terrycloth towel and lay down to rest in bed for at least

20 minutes.  If you want to sweat a bit more, then drink a large mug of pau d'arco tea prepared according to Recipe Number Four from Chapter Five right after the bath.

Such a pau d'arco bath in combination with the "Cold Killer" (Recipe Number Four, p. 52) can effectively stop a flu infection on the advance.  However, in such cases you should considerably increase the amount of pau d'arco that you drink the following three days.  It should be at least three-quarters of a liter daily, unsweetened, and between meals, as in the course of treatment.  Prepare it according to the basic recipe.

The **partial bath:** pau d'arco tea is used in a similar manner for partial baths.  If only certain regions of the body are afflicted, such as the hands or feet in fungal infections, just bathe these areas.  Use the tea, prepared doubly strong according to the basic recipe, in an undiluted form.  Leave the afflicted part of the body in the tea for about 15 to 20 minutes.  Then you can either dry it, or, if you desire an intensification of the effect, wrap it in a pre-warmed towel and leave this on for another fifteen minutes.


## Pau d'Arco in the Homeopathic Preparation

The great physician and pharmacist Samuel Hahnemann established the healing art of homeopathy almost 200 years ago.  He assumed that a medicine used by a healthy person over a longer period of time in larger amounts could produce symptoms similar to those it can cure in someone who is ill.  In Latin, this law says: "Similia similibus curantur." (Like is cured by like.) A great number of practical studies have confirmed this rule.  Furthermore, Hahnemann discovered that medications have a more profound and at the same time harmonious effect when they are potentiated, which means diluted in a specific ratio with a carrier substance such as water and then rhythmically shaken.  It would take too much time to explain this extensive system in detail, but I have included titles of some excellent literature on this topic in the appendix.

For our concerns here, it is important to know some things about the practical application of the homeopathic principle in relation to pau d'arco. In fact, you can even prepare pau d'arco yourself in a homeopathic manner. Unfortunately, according to my research this can't be acquired in an industrially manufactured form.

To make it yourself, use a dropper and several clean glass bottles holding about 50 ml (milliliters). You can get them at any pharmacy. In addition, you need some pau d'arco tea that you have prepared and boiled water that has cooled to room temperature, as well as a thick telephone book. Use the dropper to put one drop of the tea into one of the glass bottles, then fill it up with 99 drops of the boiled water. Close the bottle and hit it firmly against the telephone book 10 times. Voilà! You have just made the homeopathic remedy Pau d'Arco in the potency of (level of dilution) C1 yourself. Now take a drop from the liquid Pau d'Arco C1, put it in another little bottle, fill this in turn with 99 drops of the boiled water, close it, and again hit it 10 times against the telephone book. In this bottle you now have the homeopathic remedy Pau d'Arco in the potency of C2. Now fill it up completely with vodka and take one to five drops of the liquid several times a day under your tongue when you are ill. It works best if you don't eat or drink anything for fifteen minutes before and after taking it.

Use the homeopathic pau d'arco *only* when you are really sick and immediately stop using it when you once again feel healthy and the symptoms have disappeared. Don't take the homeopathic pau d'arco as a preventative measure and always just as drops.

Please don't make any potencies higher than C6 for administration. The competent application of higher homeopathic potencies requires appropriate training and experience. A doctor or healing practitioner who is familiar with this healing art will be able to advise you properly on it. You should always consult a specialist if you want to use homeopathic pau d'arco in potencies higher than C6 or for long than one week.

## Pau d'Arco for Pets

Some animals, as reported to me by several users, like to drink pau d'arco tea. It can be prepared for them with the same basic recipe as for humans. Otherwise, as described above, the contents of pau d'arco capsules can be mixed with the feed. By the way, together with grapefruit seed extract capsules, this is a very efficient worming treatment that doesn't strain the animal's organism. For fleas, ticks, and other parasites that like to settle in the fur and skin, you can also do a moist rub-down with pau d'arco tea in addition to internal application; or, if the animal is used to it, give it a pau d'arco bath. As a preventative measure against parasite infestation and particularly during the "tick season," simply give pau d'arco in some form once a day.

In some regions of the Andes, dogs are given pau d'arco as a preventative measure against rabies infections. Unfortunately, I don't have any detailed information about this.

## Pau d'Arco for Plants—A Research Project

Although I don't have any reports on experiences, it can be concluded from the effects of pau d'arco with a certain probability that in the case of parasitic infestation of plants, the addition of pau d'arco tea to the watering can and the spraying of the leaves and stems should actually discourage pests. If you have an inquiring mind, you can try this out.

## Pau d'Arco—For Everyday Use

**Pau d'arco as a healthy, daily beverage:** If pau d'arco is used as a pleasant-tasting, wholesome, and health-maintaining house tea, the recommended amount is one to four cups of 0.15 liters each a day according to a person's age, size, weight, state of health, and—last but not least—desire to drink it. In this form of application, the positive effects on the metabolism result less from the amounts consumed than from enjoying the tea on a *regular basis*. With the help of the delicious recipes listed in Chapter 5, pau d'arco can be prepared in new variations time and again. You can drink it both with the meals and in between. So there are a variety of ways to drink it.

By the way: If you occasionally drink more of the tea from the "divine tree" simply because it tastes so good—no problem! It has been proved that pau d'arco isn't toxic but even extensively promotes healthy well-being. This is why the Indios of South America have been using it as a daily beverage since the times of the Incas and Aztecs.

**The pau d'arco treatment**: In order to take concentrated action for the benefit of your health, the following dosage can basically be used:

Six to twelve cups of about 0.15 liters a day. Prepare according to the basic recipe in Chapter 5.

Other than when using it as a house tea, within the scope of a pau d'arco course of treatment it's better to drink the tea when your stomach is as empty as possible. Drink it either unsweetened or with just a bit of raw honey or raw sugar molasses. Avoid extreme drinking temperatures, meaning cool but not ice cold; warm but not hot. From the recipes in Chapter 5, I recommend that you select the basic preparation, as well as numbers 2, 3, 4, 7, 8, and 9. Of this, the largest portion should be prepared according to the basic recipe. The other methods of preparation are naturally not forbidden but should be enjoyed much less frequently within the scope of a course of treatment.

## Nutritional tips for the pau d'arco treatment

If you want to make the work easier for pau d'arco, you can achieve a great deal with a meaningful selection of foods.

**Avoid:**
- Pork or products containing pork
- Foods that contain preservatives, artificial dyes
- Highly heated milk products of all types
- Sodas containing sugar, sweets, cake
- Refined sugar
- Alcohol, tobacco, and other social drugs
- Adding extra salt to meals

- Foods and beverages containing excessive salt
- Packaged and canned foods
- Using the microwave and deep-fat fryer to prepare your meals
- Warming up left-overs
- Heavily fried foods
- Sausage
- White-flour products
- Vinegar made of synthetic acetic acid

**Reduce:**
- Concentrated milk products
- Eating meat in general
- Large meals—it's better to divide them into several smaller ones
- Meals after 6 p.m.
- Stress while eating
- Eating in restaurants
- Consuming beverages together with meals

**Prefer:**
- Foods from organic-ecological cultivation
- Foods that have been blanched and carefully simmered to preserve nutrients, as well as salads
- Low-sodium mineral water as a beverage
- Fish
- Fruit and vegetables
- Freshly prepared foods
- Variety in your diet
- Fresh herbs for seasoning
- Raw honey and raw sugar molasses for sweetening
- Raw milk products
- Cold-pressed oils, particularly olive oil, linseed oil, thistle oil, sunflower oil
- Salads with many plants containing chlorophyll
- Six small meals a day
- Conscious selection of foods according to your momentary appetite

- Lemon juice, or Aceto Balsamico (balsam vinegar) instead of "normal" vinegar
- Chew each bite well
- Whole-grain products
- Peace and quiet while you eat
- Food that is optically and aromatically appealing

**Tips for your lifestyle in general during a pau d'arco treatment:**
- Avoid intensive stress, as far as possible
- Take frequent walks in the fresh air
- Keep a journal on your dreams, your emotional states, and physical reactions during the treatment time.
- Think about your life and your goals that you have for the future

Caution! For serious health disorders and all symptoms that could indicate such state, you absolutely must call on a doctor. Definitely speak with your attending physician about the way you are applying pau d'arco, the dosage, and your reaction to the treatment. Many doctors who use naturopathy are already familiar with pau d'arco.

Chapter 9

# What Are Healing Reactions?

As a food supplement with a holistically beneficial effect on the organism, pau d'arco with its unique combination of active ingredients exercises a healing influence in keeping with nature on the *entire* organism. In detail, this means:

🙠 The body as a whole is detoxified. Substances capable of damaging it are more intensively eliminated or transformed into harmless substances.

*Examples of toxic substances within this context:* exhaust fumes from cars, solvents, softening agents, preservatives, pesticides, heavy metals, and residue from antibiotics and chemotherapy.

🙠 The body is thoroughly cleaned out. This means that the blood vessels, the lymph system, the cells, organs and connective tissue, as well as other areas of the organism, are cleansed of substances that, although they aren't poisonous, impede the normal vital functions. These substances are also eliminated for the most part and sometimes transformed into something more tolerable for the body.

*Examples:* proteins that can't be utilized by the metabolism may, among other things, deposited on the vessel walls or seal up the vessels as mucous; cholesterol deposits on the vessel walls; excessive salt that retains water and therefore swells up the tissue; deposits in the intestines; sugar crystals on the walls of the blood vessels in diabetics.

Through extensive removal of waste materials, illnesses that have existed and been suppressed (chronic) for a longer period of time may briefly become acute. This is the *natural course* of a healing.

*Example:* A person has had a runny nose time and again for months, as well as a sore throat and swollen tonsils with infallible regularity. A stubborn cough keeps persisting. The complaints get better sometimes, and then they return again. The cold doesn't really heal.  When pau d'arco develops its effects, an attack of fever *may* arise for several days, showing that the body's immune system is now at full speed and finally properly defending itself against the pathogens. Coughing, a runny nose, and sore throat *may* be intensified *for several days* within this context.  These manifestations actually cleanse the organism.  The expectoration removes harmful substances from the head, throat, and chest area. Sore throat and swollen tonsils indicate an active detoxification activity of the lymph system*.

In addition, through the elimination and processing of the toxins and waste materials, the following manifestations can also occur up to the completion of the internal cleansing:

- The urine is eliminated more abundantly, has an unusual coloration, and smells different than it normally does
- The stools are increasingly eliminated, appearing and smelling differently than otherwise
- There is increased sweating, and the perspiration has an unusual smell
- Coating on the tongue
- Skin reactions like rashes and pimples
- In cases of severe inner waste material accumulation, suppurations may (rarely) occur as drastic processes of elimination
- Through the strong commitment of the organism to cleansing and healing, a person may feel more tired and fatigued than otherwise for some time, having a greater need for relaxation
- The breath smells unusual or bad
- The skin becomes more oily

---

* The lymph system represents an independent vascular system within the body, which is kept flowing by the activity of the musculature.  In simple terms, this means: little movement = lymphatic congestion (lymphostasis)—much movement = promotion of the lymph flow that is so important for healing and maintenance of health.  Harmful substances are directed out of the tissue and brought to elimination through the lymphatic liquid.

- Scales appear on the scalp and the hair becomes oily more quickly
- Colds and coughs
- Diarrhea
- Temporarily lowered ability to bear emotional stress, intensified dreaming, more frequent crying, and an overall more lively expression of feelings
- Temporary swelling on lymph nodes

For holistic, natural healing, the body must use the ways it has available to it to get rid of things that strain it. It needs its strength for house-cleaning and renovating, which summarizes the meaning of the healing reactions. Please don't be afraid of them: Healing reactions occur, and they are individually different in their type and extent in every natural treatment process. This applies to homeopathy, Reiki, acupuncture, polarity, shiatsu, fasting, or hydropathic (Kneipp) treatment.

To still "play it safe," in case of doubt you should absolutely consult a doctor who works in a holistic manner. For serious illnesses and everything that could be serious, please go to the doctor before the beginning of the course of treatment in order to get the advice of a specialist.

# Chapter 10

# Catuaba, the Feel-Good Tea An Ideal Supplement to Pau d'Arco

Pau d'arco can be combined with other medicinal plants in order to achieve optimal results for certain health imbalances. An important characteristic of pau d'arco is namely that, because of its special saponins, it works like a catalyst in an herbal tea mixture to improve the effectiveness and often also the tolerance of the other components. For this reason, I have described a very interesting example of such combinations in this chapter.

## Catuaba Awakens the Joy in Life

Catuaba tea is highly valued as an aphrodisiac in Brazil. It can be said that catuaba tea is a solid component of the Brazilian culture. The rainforest plant catuaba is freely translated to mean "good tree" by the *Tupi tribe*. The tea acquired from the bark of this bush has been well-known and valued because of its animating and gastric-toning effects for centuries.

The following healing powers have traditionally been ascribed to it:

- Normalizes circulation
- Relieves spasms
- Tones the nerves
- Tranquilizes the stomach
- Relieves and heals nervous stomach complaints
- Promotes potency and libido
- Strengthens the reproductive organs in general
- Is healing for various forms of skin cancer. (Combined internal [tea] and external [decoction compress] application.)

There are no known side-effects or interactions. Catuaba tea has been used for centuries in South America.

The preparation is very similar to that of pau d'arco: 1 tablespoon for one liter of tea, boil for 5 minutes, and let draw for 15 minutes.

Catuaba tea has an aroma similar to citrus and tastes very good. It can also be dosed according to taste.

As a treatment, it's best to use it together with pau d'arco, for 14 days to three weeks, in larger amounts so that the vital spirits awaken once again. The circulation is improved throughout the entire body, particularly in the area of the pelvic organs, the nerves are calmed and can recuperate. Even many tensions are relieved.

But please note: If you drink the catuaba tea for a longer period of time in large amounts, it's great to have a vacation and best for your partner to participate in the tea-drinking treatment ...


## Catuaba Against Low Sexual Desire

According to the existing clinical studies and reports of many users, catuaba—particularly in connection with pau d'arco—appears to me to be a good, rather thrifty, and pleasant-tasting remedy against the increasingly wide-spread LSD (low sexual desire) syndrome. This illness of modern civilization, which can also be observed in animals subject to continuous stress, manifests itself in the drastic reduction of sexual desire and simultaneous increase of nervousness, tension, and excessive irritation, together with constant exhaustion and fatigue. Since a normal functioning of sexuality is also a clear gauge of the organism's health, we can assume that the LSD syndrome is a constantly overtaxed body's cry for help. The purifying, regenerating, relaxing, and nerve-strengthening effects of the combination catuaba and pau d'arco counteract this in a natural, well-tolerable, and even pleasant-tasting manner.

**Please note:** Catuaba tea is a good *dye*. If you happen to get a spot on the tablecloth or your shirt, wash it out immediately since you'll hardly be able to get it out otherwise.

In conclusion, here are two anecdotes:

In South America, people like to give breeding stallions catuaba as a "tonic."

There's a saying in Brazil: If a man up to the age of 60 fathers a child, it was him. If this happens afterwards, it was catuaba.

# Chapter 11

# The Healing Powers of Wild-Growing Plants

From the jungles, the naturally intact landscapes, come many of the most effective curative plants. There's a saying among ethnobotanists that it hardly matters what plant is studied in terms of its medical effects in the rainforest—each of them would have at least one valuable healing ability. Why do the plants of unspoiled nature have so much to offer?

In my opinion, there are two main reasons for this:

1. They grow in an environment that is optimally attuned to them. In nature, plants don't grow in monocultures. They settle with other plants species and animals that fit together with them in a particularly beneficial manner. Every hobby gardener knows that not every plant gets along with every other and takes this fact into consideration when designing his or her garden. On the other hand, there are certain plants that keep each other mutually healthy and wonderfully support each other in their growth. Certain animals also tend to fit in better with special plants in a living space—and not with others. There where nature has a free hand to do what it wants, it quickly makes sure that the optimal mixture is created. Only the intervention of human beings causes imbalances. What do we really know about the large organism covering the surface of our planet?! We are just beginning to slowly comprehend that we have much too little understanding of the complex correlations of nature. It would basically be best for us to give nature a great deal more free space so that our environment can continue—or finally begin once again—to function meaningfully.

2. Far away from industry and highways, there are hardly harmful substances that can negatively influence the metabolism of the plants. So they develop their full powers. Among other things, this can be determined in their medical effect. Many types of plants still contain their strength and healing power that has grown in their natural environment through generations until they have gradually been reduced by the systematic interbreeding, growing in plantations, cultivation and regimentation carried out by human hands.

If we believe the old European writings about the native medicinal herbs, the impression is quickly made that the healing power of plants must have also been stronger in our latitudes centuries ago. Here there were also thick primeval forests with an immensely large variety of species, although the highly "civilized" seafaring nations, the Romans and the Cathaginians, made sure that giant areas of once flourishing landscapes turned into steppe at a very early date. Three thousand years ago, the Sahara was once much, much smaller ...

There are certainly still native plants with great powers of healing in Europe and the Mediterranean region. Yet, compared with the primeval forests of Africa and South America, these tend to be in the minority.

Nevertheless, various groups have recognized this wretched state of affairs and undertaken enormous efforts for decades to once again orient the care and shaping of the landscape towards more natural principles. The trend towards foods from organic-ecological cultivation supports this movement, which has in the meantime spread throughout the world. Anyone who understands the meaning of this reorientation can personally contribute to giving nature more space in his or her own garden, by way of the city council or through citizens' initiatives.

# Chapter 12

# Nine Valuable Exercises for Activating the Immune System

As effective as medicinal plants are, people with poor health should be clearly aware that a change in their lifestyle, their way of thinking and dealing with their feelings in a harmonious, positive, and natural way may often be *the* most important help in achieving long-term healing. This is why I have compiled nine effective exercises in this chapter to help support a long-term reorientation of the way of life towards more happiness and health.

## Focusing Attention on Positive Things Time and Again (Exercise 1)

It can pretty much make a person sick when he or she surrenders to the habit of primarily perceiving the bad, burdensome, and frustrating things in life. In contrast, as also adequately demonstrated by modern medical research, a cheerful, balanced psyche supports the healing process, rejuvenates and promotes successes. Just observe how a person's posture becomes more upright, radiates more charisma, and tensed facial features relax when he or she thinks about something beautiful, completely immersing in these pleasant thoughts.

Now do your own experiment. Think of beautiful things for three minutes. How do you feel afterwards?

You can consciously tap this regenerating source of strength *since it's just a habit to mainly be aware of the negative things in life.* And habits can be changed, thank God ...

You've already taken a step in the right direction by reading this text—in the direction where healing, vitality, and success increasingly come into your life structure.

Start writing a journal. Every evening note at least ten joyful, happy, or satisfying moments that you have experienced that day. It doesn't have to be anything monumental—simply good experiences. You can't find that many? Make a thorough search because you are looking for your healing, your happiness! The more effort you make to recognize the happiness in your everyday life, the more happiness you will attract and experience. And it just happens that happy people are healthier people.

## Smiling at the Inner Organs (Exercise 2)

The Taoist exercise of *inner smiling* comes from the China of antiquity. This so effective that it's regularly employed by many hospitals in Asia as a supportive treatment for chronic ailments. In case you don't have any precise anatomical knowledge, to do this you will need a book or an illustrated table on the position and approximate appearance of the following organs: stomach, spleen, pancreas, liver, gallbladder, kidneys, heart, lungs, large intestine, small intestine, and reproductive organs.

Look for a quiet place in which you can spend about 20 minutes without being disturbed. Then set an alarm clock so you won't have to keep looking at the time.

Close your eyes and direct your attention to your body. Listen to the beat of your heart, notice the lifting and sinking of your chest as you breathe, feel the areas of your skin that have contact with what you're sitting on.

Now smile—it doesn't have just to be in your spirit! Imagine the above-mentioned organs individually and one after the other, joyfully smiling at each of them as if you are finally seeing a good friend from whom you've been separated for months.

At the conclusion of the exercise, feel the flow of your breath for a while. You can naturally also concentrate this technique on one organ or other part of your body.

## Doing Something Good for Yourself
## Every Day (Exercise 3)

No, this doesn't mean eating even more, drinking alcohol, watching TV, or smoking! Be creative. Write a list of experiences that make you happy and give yourself one of them every day. Perhaps this could be a bath in the tub with a particularly good bath oil, or perhaps it's a special film or concert that thrills your heart, or simply fifteen minutes on a park bench with a romantic view with which you pamper yourself. The important thing about this exercise is that the fulfillment of your wish depends completely on yourself! Otherwise, there will be too many excuses. However: If your partner is only too willing to massage your feet or hands now and then or go dancing with you, this naturally counts as well.

## Making Yourself a Compliment (Exercise 4)

The immune system, in terms of its strength and ability to deal with stress in relation to environmental influences, is dependent upon how much we like ourselves. The more *self-love*, *self-respect*, and *self-confidence* we have, the more beneficial the conditions for our body's own well-functioning defense system. There is a simple way to help you use these positive influences for your own well-being. Make yourself a compliment every day—two or three are even better. It doesn't even matter what the compliment is for. It doesn't have to be anything great or enormously important. It should just be something that you've done well, something that is lovable about yourself, or something that deserves respect or recognition.

This exercise is most effective when you do it in front of a mirror, look yourself in the eyes, and smile at yourself. Don't worry, it's only you! Learn to value and love yourself more every day by expressly recognizing the good in yourself through compliments. Your body will soon thank you for it and your peace of mind as well. If it's hard for you to praise and smile at yourself, you can be comforted by knowing that a lot of other people feel the same way. Why else would there be so many acute and chronic health disorders today that are based on weakness of the immune system?! Keep practicing every day and go through your resistance! Do it for your happiness and your health!

P.S.: Expand this exercise as soon as possible by giving three people around you a compliment every day. When we acknowledge others, we will also be more appreciated ourselves.

## Seek the Encounter with God (Exercise 5)

The ancient medical texts from China emphasized that the greatest healing power for human beings lies in the attunement with the divine. Perhaps this is why chronic diseases occur significantly less frequently among the religious community of the Mormons in the USA, for example.

You don't have to be a member of a church or a sect, or even believe in God, to experience the healing, pleasant power of an encounter with the divine. Simply try the following exercise; this will convince you of the usefulness of my advice!

First, learn to pray. No, I don't mean the usual requests that go "up there" for material things, a partner, or prompt recuperation. An effective prayer functions in another way— it shouldn't be too focused towards a direct benefit.

*The less a person concretely expects,*
*The more life can give him!*

Take several minutes of time every day in which you can retreat and have no one make any demands on you. It really doesn't have to be any more than that. Close your eyes. Then imagine that somewhere above you there is something from which everything in our world has been made and to which everything will return again at some time. Once again: You don't have to believe in it. Just simply carry out this exercise carefully on a regular basis for several weeks! Then also imagine coming closer to a being, the source of all life and therefore also of health. Pay attention to your feelings during this encounter, but don't expect anything in particular. Be open to whatever happens. Keep your attention focused on this until the end of the exercise. You can set an alarm clock so you don't have to look at the time. I personally like to do this exercise before I go to sleep. No one disturbs me then and I take the pleasant experience of encountering the *Highest Being* along with me in my dreams.

If you want to do more, then occasionally go to an old church, power place, or pilgrimage site. Feel the special atmosphere of these places, and try to surrender to it. It doesn't matter if you feel somewhat strange and out of place at first. You soon won't want to miss these—in the truest sense—uplifting moments in your life.

By the way: If significant personalities like Mahatma Gandhi, Albert Einstein, Johann Wolfgang von Goethe, and John F. Kennedy have bestowed so much importance on prayer and approaching the spiritual power on a regular basis—why shouldn't you also make successful use of this simple help that is without cost and accessible for everyone?

## Forgiving Yourself (Exercise 6)

Forgiveness, deep and sincere forgiveness, frees the soul from causes of constant conflict, from tensions that bind the powers of the body and mind urgently needed in the present. Thoughts of revenge and unforgiving behavior damage the striving for happiness and health. Once you have realized that the past is no longer changeable—that it has *passed*—you can learn from your experiences. Then you can better and more easily master the challenges of the present. Make a list of ways of behavior, actions, thoughts, and words for which you haven't been able to forgive yourself, for which you are ashamed. Become clear about wanting to deal with them more constructively in the future. For each point, write down the first steps of how you can learn this and keep your positive intentions in mind. Set up a timetable for the reorientation and monitor how you are following it every day.

Then take some minutes for a small but very effective mental exercise:

- Visualize how you have always been at loggerheads with yourself up to now because you have behaved differently than the ethical standards that you set for yourself and how you have unnecessarily strained the good relationships with fellow beings who perhaps were quite important to you. Decide to consciously create your future in a different way from now! You are a being capable of learning and become as you want to be: loved, valued, and respected by your fellow beings and yourself!
- Now let your thoughts travel into the future situations, in which you behave in the new, more constructive ways that you have decided upon for yourself. Spend some time enjoying the pleasant feeling that is created when you get the positive feedback of your surrounding world for the maturing of your personality. Congratulate yourself on the decision that you have made and which you have stood by until the change has been completely made. Now you can be full of self-respect as you look in the mirror and say to yourself: "I've made mistakes. I'm allowed to do this because I'm a human being. I've done my best to learn from them and have changed myself, becoming more mature. I did what I could in order to grow!" Now spend a moment in these feelings arising within you.
- Take a few deep breaths, and stretch your body. Open your eyes in the awareness that you have taken the first step in the right direction. Now get up and do whatever is necessary to completely turn your decision into action.

By the way, it may be helpful to speak the course of the exercise on a cassette and let yourself be guided by it. This will free your mind for the experience.

## Forgiving Someone Else (Exercise 7)

As important as it is to forgive ourselves, it's just as important to forgive others who have hurt us. On the one hand, you may possible suffer the most when you are filled with wrath and harbor thoughts of revenge against certain fellow beings. This is because it ties up much of your emotional energy that is urgently needed to the full extent, not only for mental activities but also for the healthy control of your bodily functions. On the other hand, through the constant conscious or unconscious discord, you are in a continual state of tension and direct your attention to largely sorrowful situations of your past that you have no possibility of changing. This means that you can use the diverse possibilities of being happy and successful in the present only to a limited extent. You continue to be in your own way.

Stop doing this! Right now! What you have experienced is bad enough—you don't have to make it even worse by continuing to emotionally cling to the associated anger and injuries until never-never day. Decide for your own good, for your happiness, *to finally close the files on it!* Perhaps you still don't understand the other person—try it! Perhaps it's not clear to you how you contributed to the escalation of the situation—find this out! Perhaps there's still too much anger within you to be able to forgive—then read Exercise Number 8 and relieve yourself systematically of your aggressions. Make the positive effects of the sorrowful situation clear to yourself. What, there aren't any? That can't be—in thousands of personal consultations in my practice, I have always been able to conclude that people who are sorely tried by fate in the difficult situations that they've experienced have gained much human maturity, the ability to deal with things, knowledge—and often also sympathy and tolerance.

In one sentence: People who have gone through a great deal often know more about life!

It's not so easy to put one over on them. Look at your past with this perspective. You don't need to love the other person who has hurt you so much. But, with the help of the tips in this exercise, you can develop so much clarity in relation to this experience that you can sincerely forgive him or her. And you will do this in the certainty of having done yourself the greatest favor.

In conclusion, here is one bit of advice: It may be that you have a hard time in forgiving because you consciously or unconsciously are afraid that something terrible like this could happen to you again. *Particularly because of this*, you will learn from the experience, as in this exercise. Armed with the new expanded consciousness, in case there is a next time you will be able to get out of the way in time or be able to take much better care of yourself.

## Relieve Yourself of Aggressions on a Regular Basis without Hurting Yourself or Others (Exercise 8)

Every day we experience so many things: things that are beautiful and burdensome, harmonious and frustrating moods. It frequently isn't possible to immediately express our anger in an appropriate way. This is why it can accumulate and slowly start to poison the life of our soul. We suddenly notice that we angrily shout at someone who actually isn't at fault. When there are enough accumulated aggressions, they can even promote an increased tendency towards accidents. We then endanger not only our own health but also the health of other people who really aren't responsible for the old frustration within us.

A simple exercise can help you free yourself of the inner tensions accumulated during everyday life. Done on a regular basis in a harmless manner, this is even good for your body. However, you need two things to help you do this: a sandbag and a pair of boxing gloves. You can get these items at a sporting goods store. Look for a place in your home where the sandbag can swing freely and then you can get started ...

Establish 10 to 15 minutes of practice time every evening, right after you get home. For the first four to five minutes, just hit the training device with your hands, which are protected by the boxing gloves, in a relaxed way in order to warm up. This is how you can protect your body from injuries based on sudden intensive strain. Tendons and muscles can take a lot of strain—when they are warmed up. Then you can "really go at it." But don't overdo it. Take it easy at the start. Imagine what you want while you do this. It's not going to hurt anyone. To the contrary: You will soon discover that it's pleasantly easier to be relaxed in dealing with the many difficult people around you. In this way, you will turn more and more opponents into friends. In addition, it has been proved that people who reduce their frustration in a meaningful way on a regular basis can physically and mentally take much more strain in times of crisis, therefore dealing with stress much more successfully. At the same time, the self-healing powers of the body will function more efficiently, you breathe more deeply, and the organism also has much more vital energy available to it, which is a further important effect of this exercise, particularly in correlation with the topics treated in this book.

## Discover the Diversity of Your Emotional World (Exercise 9)

You probably remember this from your teenager years: listening to music and immersing yourself in a great variety of emotions, simply daydreaming in a relaxed way. Nature has been very wise in structuring things so that people become deeply receptive to music particularly during puberty, therefore getting to know and living out the great spectrum of their emotions in such an entertaining, pleasant way. Unfortunately, most people don't take this simple and very effective method of *mental hygiene* along into adult existence. Too bad—a great portion of life's quality gets lost as a result! In addition, being occupied with our emotions provides us with an expanded *emotional consciousness*, which can considerably improve and intensify our harmonious contacts with fellow beings. Surrendering to the flow of our feelings on a regular basis relieves the mind and body of inner tensions, releases additional energies, and even promotes creativity and healthy self-confidence. These are all qualities that beneficially influence chronic afflictions and have been successfully used in many places by doctors working holistically as a supportive therapy.

What can you do to now become more familiar with your world of feelings and let your emotions flow in a healthy way? Quite simple: Make an advance selection of some music pieces for one week at a time. Go ahead and get advice at specialized music stores. Try out something new. When listening to the music, pay attention to changes in your feelings. Which images, emotions, associations arise during which songs? How does your body feel? How does it feel to you during each piece of music? Keep a small notebook with you and write down your inner experiences with the music several times a day. In no case should you make this exercise complicated and elaborate! Simply be sure that you are surrounded by music at every possible opportunity. It's important to listen to it consciously time and again, and then briefly feel what's going on inside yourself. Write down the key words about what you perceive inside yourself.

Here's another little anecdote: You are certainly familiar with the constant background music in department stores with which the "esteemed customers" are influenced to more willingly buy things and increase sales, and you have probably also heard that cows give more milk and are less stressed when they hear harmonious, relaxing music. Hearing is our sense that is most strongly connected with the emotional world. Researchers like the famous musicologist *Joachim Ernst Behrendt* have demonstrated this extensively and conclusively in their work. Music apparently also influences the state of the human psyche. So use this knowledge for yourself and increase your well-being and state of health in this agreeable way. In China and India, there has been music composed directly for therapeutic purposes for centuries, so why shouldn't we here in the West employ this knowledge of the inner life for ourselves?*

---

* In the Appendix V there are a number of music productions listed that have been specifically composed and recorded in Asia for the supportive treatment of certain ailments.

# Epilog

While reading this book, you may have had the impression that pau d'arco is a type of miracle drug, an infallible healing remedy—but this certainly isn't the case. There are no infallible healing remedies and there probably never will be. In addition, I don't want to create the impression in any way that everyone can now cure themselves alone of the most serious diseases without consulting a doctor. Pau d'arco is wonderfully suited as a house tea for the prevention of many afflictions and can contribute a great deal to curing various health problems. But despite this, anyone who has something that could possibly be a serious illness should consult the appropriate doctor about it. Healing must be learned and the layperson can all too easily overlook something important, wrongly evaluate a symptom, or do too much or too little of a good thing.

For my part, I have consulted doctors, healing practitioners, and psychotherapists who are open to their patients taking responsibility for themselves, supporting their initiative for self-treatment in a justifiable manner and to an appropriate extent. I also like to recommend these professionals to participants in my seminars and to clients in my personal consultation practice.

Any physician who is trained in naturopathy will quickly learn to value the manifold healing powers of pau d'arco—in case he or she hasn't yet become familiar with it and desires to include pau d'arco in the medical treatment according to whether it's basically appropriate for the case. It's up to us, hopefully as responsible citizens, to support the physicians who take us and our striving for health seriously. Those who go to a doctor just because they've always gone to him or her or because the doctor has been willing to report them sick without a real reason should take the time to consider if they are really doing the best thing for themselves. We have the choice—in every respect. And the more people who deal with it wisely, the more quickly our health system will change over to holistic medicine, and the better the chances will be for curing chronic afflictions.

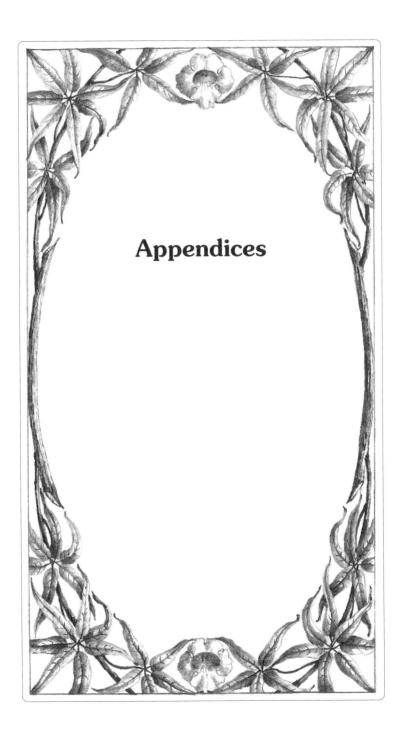

# Appendices

# Appendix I

# The Most Important Information at a Glance

## Preparation (basic recipe)

For 1 liter, add 1 to 2 tablespoons of pau d'arco tea in bubbly, boiling water and let boil for 5 minutes. Then let draw while covered for another 15 – 20 minutes without heat. Pour the finished tea into a storage container through a tea strainer or—even better—a linen cloth.

## Application as house tea

Enjoy the various pau d'arco preparations according to your desire for them on a regular basis. However, the emphasis should be on the basic recipe.

## Treatment application

Drink six to twelve cups of about 0.15 liters each day, at best on an empty stomach. The drinking temperature shouldn't be much higher than the body temperature. You can also use it cooled.

## Side effects

Of the pau d'arco species available on the international market, it's known that **very high** doses of the tea or its extracts can sometimes lead to a slight itching of the skin and a bit of rash. According to all the information I've received, both manifestations can be seen as harmless and immediately disappear when the daily administered dose is reduced. There are no types of unfavorable consequences known.

In a few species of the lapacho tree, the inner bark contains a high portion of tannins. In case of frequent contact, they may irritate the mucous membranes of the stomach, the area of the mouth and throat and the esophagus. **However, this happens *only* when the tea is used at a very hot temperature.** Even at body temperature, there are no types of problems, and this certainly also applies to the cooled tea. Although few of these types of pau d'arco tea are on the market, for safety's sake you should still pay attention to the drinking temperature—see the section on "Treatment application." You can also add a bit of milk or cream to the tea.

## Contraindications

In my research I haven't been able to find any for the species of pau d'arco available on the international market.

## Interactions with medications or herbal preparations

Despite careful research, I have not been able to find any reports on negative interactions of pau d'arco with medications. To the contrary, pau d'arco can be combined particularly well with other herbal remedies because it is able to directly and indirectly increase the health-promoting effects of the accompanying preparations through the metabolism.

**What pau d'arco can do:**

- Eliminate toxins, waste materials, heavy metals, etc. Eliminate amalgam during and after the teeth have been repaired.
- Normalize and strengthen the functions of the inner organs such as the liver, kidneys, and spleen, as well as the digestion.
- Directly kill some disease-causing types of fungus, and indirectly destroy the others by stimulating the body's own immune system.
- Directly kill viruses, bacteria, and parasites and additionally help the body protect itself against the infections and infestations, as well as protecting itself against becoming ill again, by extensively stimulating its own defense system.
- Comprehensively strengthen the organism.
- Cure depressions based on metabolic imbalances (for example: disorders of the liver function resulting from previous chemotherapy or long-term use of psychopharmacological agents).
- Improve the circulation.
- Inhibit and dissolve tumor of all kinds.
- Exercise a healing influence on leukemia.
- Overcome anemia.
- Build up the body's own immune system.
- Eliminate deposits in the blood vessels.
- Stimulate a sluggish metabolism.
- Normalize the sugar metabolism.
- Exercise a healing influence on diabetes and the delayed damage resulting from this disease or preventing the latter.
- Favorably influence the course of chronic diseases like multiple sclerosis, Parkinson's disease, arthritis, and rheumatism.
- Give the nervous system of greater ability to deal with stress and strain.
- Strengthening and normalize the sexual functions.
- Relieve pain.

- Favorably influence migraines and other states of chronic pain.
- Heal skin rashes, wounds, and suppurations.
- Help heal inflammations of all types.
- Have a diuretic effect.
- Calm the psyche.
- Relieve congestion of all types within the body.
- Strengthen the heart and circulation.
- Promote healthy sleep.
- Soothe the fears that arise from metabolic problems.
- Boost the natural function of the sweat glands.
- Exercise a calming influence on the nervous system.

**Be sure to pay attention to the following when buying pau d'arco:**
- The cut bark should have a reddish-brown appearance.
- Cardboard and paper are best-suited as packaging material. Longer storage in certain types of plastic at higher surrounding temperatures can reduce the healing effects of the pau d'arco tea.
- The dealer should be able to give exact information as to the species of lapacho plant from which the bark for the tea that he or she is selling originated.
- Give preference to the types of pau d'arco that tend to be more expensive. Then the chance is actually greater that you will be getting high-quality merchandise.
- In case of doubt, if a good therapeutic effect is important to you, stick with merchandise from brandname manufacturers that have been involved with pau d'arco for a longer period of time and can also provide exact information about it.

# What's in pau d'arco tea?

The following chemical analysis refers to how many fractions of a milligram are contained of a nutritionally important substance per milligram of the pau d'arco bark powder ...

| | | |
|---|---|---|
| Traces of | arsenic | (mg./mg.) |
| 0.083 | calcium | (mg./mg.) |
| 0.0326 | caloric value | (cal./mg.) |
| 0.00261 | carbohydrates | (mg./mg.) |
| 0.816 | chromium | (mg./mg.) |
| 0.000009 | cobalt | (mg./mg.) |
| 0.000151 | indigestible roughage | (mg./mg.) |
| 0.152 | digestible plant fibers | (mg./mg.) |
| 0.494 | fat | (mg./mg.) |
| 0.005 | iron | (mg./mg.) |
| traces of | lead | (mg./mg.) |
| 0.00081 | manganese | (mg./mg.) |
| 0.000027 | mercury | (mg./mg.) |
| 0.0000057 | phosphorus | (mg./mg.) |
| 0.00012 | potash | (mg./mg.) |
| 0.00185 | proteins | (mg./mg.) |
| 0.096 | riboflavin | (mg./mg.) |
| traces of | selenium | (mg./mg.) |
| 0.000002 | silicon | (mg./mg.) |
| 0.000084 | sodium | (mg./mg.) |
| traces of | thiamine | (mg./mg.) |
| trace of | tin | (mg./mg.) |
| 0.0000037 | vitamin A | (IU/mg.) |
| 0.00708 | vitamin C | (mg./mg.) |
| 0.000181 | zinc | (mg./mg.) |

*And here is the more easily digestible summary:*
Pau d'arco contains a series of substances that kill pathogens and parasites, as well as being capable of healing cancer. In addition, it contains a great deal of iron and calcium, including an average comparable amount of selenium. The content of magnesium, manganese, vitamin C, and zinc is min-

imal. Furthermore, there are traces of barium, gold, potassium, copper, molybdenum, sodium, nickel, phosphorus, silver, and strontium, as well as vitamin A and B-complex. If you are wondering why there are somewhat more components listed in this summary than above, this is because I have evaluated various further analyses, which were in part constructed according to the search for different substances.

## The chemical composition of pau d'arco bark powder in relation to the organic compounds

Various coumarins and saponins:
the flavonoid 4', 7-dihydroxyflavone-7-0-rutin.
Moreover ...

- 0.003% 2-acetalgaphtol (2,3-b)furan-4,9-dion, benzo(b)furan-6-aldehyde (=6-formylbenzo(b)furan,
- 0.007% (-)-6.8-dihydroxy-3-methyl-3,4-dihydroisocoumarin(=(-)-6-hydroxymellcin),
- 0.004%(-)-2,3-dihydro-2(1'methylethenyl)naphtho(2,3-b)furan-4,9-dion(=(-)-dehydro-iso-a-lapachon),
- 0.03% 3,4-dimethoxybenyaldehyde(0 veratric aldehyde),
- 0.13% 3,4-dimethoxybenzoic acid (veratric acid),
- 0.003% 2,2-dimethylnaphtho(2,3-b)pyran-5,10-dion (= dehydro-a-lapachon),
- < 0.001% 8-hydroxy-2-acetylnaphtho(2,3-b)furan-4,9-dion,
- <0.001% 5-hydroxy-2-acetylnaphtho(2,3-b)furan-4,9-dion,
- 0.001% 5-hydroxy-2,3-dihydro-2-.(1'methylethenyl)naphtho-(2,3-b)furan-4,9-dion (= 5-hydroxydehydro-iso-a-lapachon),
- <0.001% 2-hydroxy-3-(3',3'-dimethyallyl)naphtho-1,4-dion (= lapachol),
- < 0.001% (-)-5-hydroxy-2-(1'-hydroxyethyl) naphtho(2,3-b)furan-4,9-dion, <
- 0.001% (+/-)-8-hydroxy-2-(1'-hydroxyethyl)naphtho(2,3-b)furan-4,9-dion,
- 0.006% (+)-2-(1'-hydroxyethyl)naphtho(2,3-b)furan-4,9-dion, and
- 0.001% 3,4,5-trimethoxybenzoic acid (= eudesmic acid), 0.02% 4-hydroxybenzoic acid, 0.02% 4-hydroxy-3-methoxybenzoic acid (= vanillic acid),

# Scientific studies in the effectiveness of catuaba (Erythroxylum catuaba)

Manabe H., et.al. "Effects of Catuaba extracts on microbial and HIV infection," *In Vivo*, 6:2, March-April 1992.
catuaba works on the psyche like "a few hours in a hammock at the Copa Cabana." Go ahead and try it out yourself.
Graf E., et.al. "Alkaloids from Erythroxylum vacciniifolium Martius, II: The structures of catuabine A, B, and C," *Arch Pharm* (Weinheim), 311:2, February 1978.
Agar J.T., et.al. "Alkaloids of the genus Erythroxylum. Part 1. E. monogynum Roxb. roots," *Journal of the Chemical Society* (Perkin 1), 14, 1976: 1550-8.
Graf E., et.al. "Alkaloids from Erythroxylum vaccinifolium Martius, I: Isolation of catuabine A, B, and C," *Arch Pharm* (Weinheim), 310: 12, Dec. 1977: 1005-10.

One study should be described extensively at this point because it shows further important healing effects of catuaba:

"Effects of Catuaba extracts on microbial and HIV infection," Manabe H.; Sakagami, H.; Ishizone, H.; Kusano, H.; Fujimaki, M.; Wada, C.; Komatsu, N.,: Nakashima, H.; Murakami, T.; Yamamoto, N. *In Vivo*, 6:2, March-April 1992: 161-5.

With an alkaloid solution of extracts from Catuaba casca (erythorxylum catuaba Arr. Cam.), laboratory mice were effectively protected from an otherwise deadly infection of *Escherichia coli* and *Staphylococcus aureus*. The extracts clearly obstructed distinctly recognizable AIDS viruses from destroying cells. A large part of this effect was achieved through the extracts strengthening the cells to such a degree that the HIV pathogens could no longer penetrate them. The results of this clinical study indicate that catuaba extracts could have a protective effect in terms of HIV infection.

According to reports of experiences that I have received, many people quickly experience a relaxed, pleasant mood after the enjoyment of several cups of catuaba tea. However, intoxicating effects or even manifestations of addiction have never been observed. According to my experience, catuaba works on the psyche like „a few hours in a hammock at the Copa Cabana." Go ahead and try it out yourself. Catuaba has a pleasant taste, doesn't hurt you in any way, and ... certainly can do you some good!

# Appendix II

# Clinical Studies on Pau d'Arco

Anesini C., Perez C.: Catedra de Farmacologia, Facultad de Odontologia, Universidad de Buenos Aires, Argentina. "Screening of plants used in Argentine folk medicine for antimicrobial activity," *Journal Ethnopharmacol*, 39:2, June 1993: 119-28.

Binutu O.A., et al. "Antimicrobial potentials of some plant species of the Bignoniaceae family," *Afr J Med Sci*, September 1994.

Ueda S., et al. "Production of anti-tumour-promoting furanonaphthoquinones in Tabebuia avellanedae cell cultures," *Phytochemistry*, May 1994.

Grazziotin, J.D., et al. "Phytochemical and analgesic investigation of Tabebuia chrysotricha," *J Ethnopharmacol*, June 1992.

Vida-Tessier AM, et al. "Lipophilic quinones of the trunk wood of Tabebuia serratifolia. (Vahl.) Nichols," *Ann Pharm Fr*, 1988.

Rao M.M., et al. "Plant anticancer agents. XII. Isolation and structure elucidation of new cytotoxic quinones from Tabebuia cassinoides," *J Nat Prod*, September-October 1982.

Joshi K.C., et al. "Chemical examination of the roots of Tabebuia," *Planta Med*, May 1977.

Santana C.F. de, et al. "Antitumoral and toxicological properties of extracts of bark and various wood components of Pau d'arco (Tabebuia avellanedae)," *Rev Inst Antibiot* (Recife), December 1968.

# Appendix III

# More Extensive Reading

Jones, Kenneth (1995). *Pau d'Arco—Immune Power from the Rain Forest.* Rochester, Vermont: Healing Arts Press. An excellent study of pau d'arco, presented in an academic manner.

Pelton, R. and Overholser, L. (1994): *Alternatives in Cancer Therapy.* Toronto, Ontario: Fireside.

Walters, R. (1993) Options: *The Alternative Cancer Therapy Book.* Garden City Park, New York: Avery Publishing Group Inc.

Wead, Bill (1985). *Second Opinion.*

# Appendix IV

# Press Comments on Pau d'Arco

Anonymous (1993). "Questionable Methods of Cancer Management: "Nutritional" Therapies," *Ca: A Cancer Journal for Clinicians*, 43(5): 309-319.

Awang, D.V.C. (1988). "Commercial Taheebo Lacks Active Ingredient," *Canadian Pharmaceuticals Journal*, 121(5): 323-326.

Block, J.B. et al. (1974). "Early Clinical Studies with Lapachol (NSC-11905)," *Cancer Chemotherapy Reports* (2), 4: 27-28.

Girard, M. et al. (1988). "Naphthoquinone Constituents of Tabebuia Species," *Journal of Natural Products*, 51: 1023-1024.

Oswald, Edward H. (1993/94). "Lapacho," *British Journal of Phytotherapy*, Vol. 3, N. 3.

Rao, K.V. (1974). "Quinone Natural Products: Streptonigrin (NSC-4 5383) and Lapachol (NSC-11905) Structure-Activity Relationships," *Cancer Chemotherapy Reports* (2),4: 11-17.

# Appendix V

# Music that Supports Healing and Well-Being

For general relaxation, meditation, and listening to after a pau d'arco whole-body bath:

- Reiki (Merlin's Magic)
- Reiki-Light Touch (Merlin's Magic)
- Angel Helpers (Merlin's Magic)
- Desire for Love (Bach)

**Rhythmic Music for Increasing Vitality and for Expressive Dance:**
- Dynamic Dancing (Power of Movement)

**Healing Music from China:**
- Hypertension
- Intestinal Ulceration
- Headache
- Dysmenorrhea
- Constipation
- Climacteric Syndrome
- Cancer
- Stroke
- Coronary Arteriosclerosis
- Sleeping

---

All of these titles are distributed by Lotus Light Publications. Each title represents a CD.

# Appendix VI

# Commented Bibliography

## Relaxation, Personality Development, and Activation of the Body's Own Self-Healing Powers ...

*Complete Reiki Handbook.* How Reiki, the art of creating relaxation and self-healing by laying on the hands, can be practically applied. By Walter Lübeck, Lotus Light Publications.

*Reiki—Way of the Heart.* The Reiki method as a way of developing the personality. By Walter Lübeck, Lotus Light Publications.

*Reiki—For First Aid.* Specially compiled treatment patterns for harmonizing more than 40 different health problems; with extensive tips on nutrition. By Walter Lübeck, Lotus Light Publications.

*The Secrets of Loving Touch.* These gentle body exercises can have a harmonizing effect on the soul. By Frank Benedikter, Lotus Light Publications.

## Homeopathy ...

*Homeopathic Medicine Today.* Sets out the early history of homeopathy, its development in many countries—in particular its role in the United States. With detailed examinations of the homeopathic remedies, principles and techniques of prescribing, and methods of treatment. By Trevor Cook, Keats Publishing.

*Repertory of the Homeopathic Materia Medica.* Broadens one's understanding to have a better knowledge of the guiding principles of repertorising the so many remedies of our materia medica and finding out the exact similimum without much searching and consulting. By J.T. Kent, B. Jain Publishing LTD.

## Sensible Nutrition ...

*Aryurvedic Cooking for Westerners.* Western recipes that utilizes Ayurvedic principles. For people who want to practice Ayurvedic health practices in the West. By Amadea Morningstar, Lotus LIght Publications.

*Ayurveda: Life of Balance.* A complete and authoritative manual on the Vedic principles of health and nutrition. It will be of great benefit to the layperson and professional alike. By Maya Tiwari, Healing Arts Press.

*The Ayurvedic Cookbook.* Finest introduction to the use of Ayurveda in your kitchen. Wonderful recipes, easy to prepare, tasty and nutritious. By A. Morningstar and U. Desai, Lotus Light Publications.

## Spiritual Consciousness and Holistic Personality Development ...

*Ayurveda and the Mind.* The first book published in the West that explores specifically the psychological aspect of this great system: How to heal our minds on all levels from subconscious to the superconscious, along with the role of diet, impressions, mantra, meditation, yoga and many other methods to create wholeness. By Dr. David Frawley, Lotus Light Publications.

*Bhagavad Gita.* "The accomplishment in philosophy of Shankara in a short life of thirty-two years" was first made available to the world in 20 volumes, published in 1910. Edited by Parmesnwari Prasad Khetan, Sa Divine Life Trust

# The Author—Walter Lübeck

Walter Lübeck, born on February 17, 1960 (Aquarius, Sagittarius Ascendent) lives in Weserbergland/Germany, a mystical landscape with many ancient power places that inspire him both personally and professionally. He has been inter-

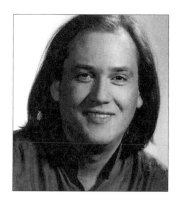

ested in esotericism, parapsychology, and methods of alternative healing since his youth.

The abundant results of his research are documented in fifteen books, which have been translated into eleven languages, and diverse articles in specialized magazines.

Walter Lübeck orients himself toward three spiritual principles: support of individual responsibility, development of the ability to love, and consciousness expansion. His goal is the concrete betterment of the quality daily life through spiritual knowledge and contributing toward bringing human beings, God, and nature into greater harmony.

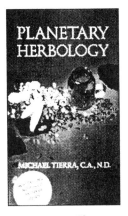

# Sources of Supply:

*The following companies have an extensive selection of useful products and a long track-record of fulfillment. They have natural body care, aromatherapy, flower essences, crystals and tumbled stones, homeopathy, herbal products, vitamins and supplements, videos, books, audio tapes, candles, incense and bulk herbs, teas, massage tools and products and numerous alternative health items across a wide range of categories.*

## WHOLESALE:

*Wholesale suppliers sell to stores and practitioners, not to individual consumers buying for their own personal use. Individual consumers should contact the RETAIL supplier listed below. Wholesale accounts should contact with business name, resale number or practitioner license in order to obtain a wholesale catalog and set up an account.*

### Lotus Light Enterprises, Inc.

P O Box 1008 PD
Silver Lake, WI 53170 USA
414 889 8501 (phone)
414 889 8591 (fax)
800 548 3824 (toll free order line)

---

## RETAIL:

*Retail suppliers provide products by mail order direct to consumers for their personal use. Stores or practitioners should contact the wholesale supplier listed above.*

### Internatural

33719 116th Street PD
Twin Lakes, WI 53181 USA
800 643 4221 (toll free order line)
414 889 8581 office phone
WEB SITE: www.internatural.com

Web site includes an extensive annotated catalog of more than 7000 products that can be ordered "on line" for your convenience 24 hours a day, 7 days a week.